White
Blood

Personal journeys with childhood leukaemia

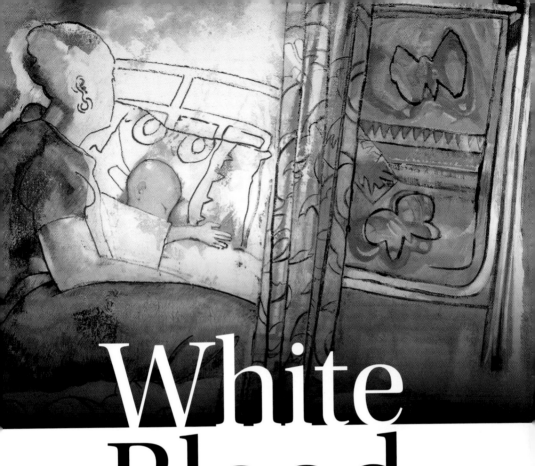

White
Blood

Personal journeys with childhood leukaemia

Editor

Mel Greaves
The Institute of Cancer Research, UK

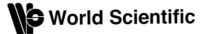
World Scientific

NEW JERSEY · LONDON · SINGAPORE · BEIJING · SHANGHAI · HONG KONG · TAIPEI · CHENNAI

Published by

World Scientific Publishing Co. Pte. Ltd.

5 Toh Tuck Link, Singapore 596224

USA office: 27 Warren Street, Suite 401-402, Hackensack, NJ 07601

UK office: 57 Shelton Street, Covent Garden, London WC2H 9HE

British Library Cataloguing-in-Publication Data
A catalogue record for this book is available from the British Library.

WHITE BLOOD

For photocopying of material in this volume, please pay a copying fee through the Copyright Clearance Center, Inc., 222 Rosewood Drive, Danvers, MA 01923, USA. In this case permission to photocopy is not required from the publisher.

ISBN-13 978-981-279-039-2
ISBN-10 981-279-039-X
ISBN-13 978-981-279-040-8 (pbk)
ISBN-10 981-279-040-3 (pbk)

Typeset by Stallion Press
Email: enquiries@stallionpress.com

Printed in Singapore by Mainland Press Pte Ltd

CONTENTS

PREFACE

The death of any child is a tragedy; a promise of life stolen. A child suffering from and then dying of cancer seems hideously cruel. There was a time in Europe when the loss of an infant or child was commonplace due to endemic infections or malnutrition. This still happens, disgracefully so, on a prodigious scale in less developed regions of the planet. But here, with social and economic advances over the past century or so, these ravages of early life have been driven back and what comes to the fore is something that somehow seems far less "natural" and more insidious — cancers, of which leukaemia is the most common. Fifty years ago, for any child, a diagnosis of leukaemia was literally a death sentence and there was near universal pessimism in the medical community over any prospect for effective treatment. But today, some 80% or more of children are cured of leukaemia — by artful combinations of drugs and chemotherapy. Legitimately, this is widely regarded as one of the real triumphs of modern medicine and science. This extraordinary turnaround did not happen overnight and its slow incremental success is a testament to courage, persistence, belief and ingenuity. But it is not, or not yet, an unmitigated triumph. Up to 20% of patients still succumb to the disease, more still in countries that lack access to state of the art diagnostic and therapeutic tools. And for children to achieve sustained remissions and likely cure, there is a two to three year ordeal of toxic treatment, obnoxious side effects and some risk of long term collateral damage. The treatment, though efficacious, is, in biological terms, still crude: effectively, blanket bombing of a target by a blind marksman. And for the parents of such children, there is the passive agony of watching the child you adore, teeter on the edge of an abyss. So much has been achieved but so much remains to be done. Fortunately, the remarkable advances in genetics, cell and molecular biology over the past two decades have unravelled the underlying mechanistic faults in DNA and cells that cause the disease. This lays the foundation to move forward so that we can deliver more targeted, less toxic therapy and ultimately unravel causes of leukaemia.

Embedded in the saga of childhood leukaemia are some extraordinary stories of human endeavour and resilience which are best told as personal narratives. In this book, we venture to compile perspectives of a kind that rarely go hand in hand. We portray the experience of childhood leukaemia as journeys taken by a clinician, a biologist, a child psychologist, a patient, and the parents of children with leukaemia. It might be considered incongruous, or even insensitive, to place alongside each other tales of hard-nosed laboratory science and personal grief. We hope not, but judge for yourself. There is also an issue of whether the particular stories told are "typical", whether it be that of the clinician or parent, etc. They are, we feel, indeed representative but at the same time, unique and special. The only alternative would have been to have multiple versions. This we feel would have been at the expense of real engagement and impact.

We hope these stories will give some comfort to families faced with a diagnosis of leukaemia in a child and for others, more fortunate, we offer them as windows into a world that can hardly be imagined as well as a celebration of the human spirit and how ordinary people deal with extraordinary circumstances.

The narratives are illustrated with evocative paintings on childhood leukaemia by a remarkable artist, Susan Macfarlane. Sadly, Susan died in 2002 and we are grateful to her sons, Euan and Angus Mackay, for their permission to reproduce some of her extraordinary paintings here, all of which derive from the exhibition 'Living with Leukaemia', commissioned by Dr. Geoffrey Farrer-Brown. The descriptions of the paintings in the legends below each image are, appropriately, in Susan's own words.

This book is dedicated to Georgie, and to other children who, like her, didn't make it through.

Mel Greaves
London

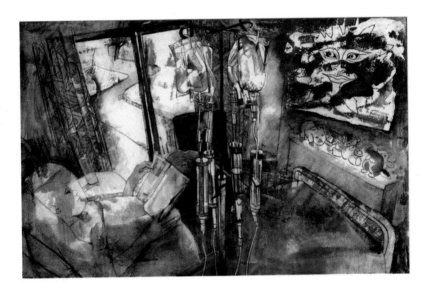

'*Waiting*' by Susan Macfarlane.

The girl reads patiently in bed during a period of transfusion with red blood cell and platelet concentrates during the recovery stage following bone marrow transplant. She is shown in an isolated cubicle at the Bone Marrow Transplant Unit where patients remain 3–5 weeks after marrow transplant. "*The patient wanted to know just what I was doing and hoped she would be able to come to the exhibition, in due course.*" Oil on Canvas. 76 × 116 cm. (Courtesy of Euan and Angus Mackay and Dr Geoffrey Farrer-Brown).

LIST OF FIGURES

LIST OF PAINTINGS

THE AUTHORS' BIOSKETCHES

A Paediatrician

Donald Pinkel is a Professor Emeritus of Pediatrics at the University of Texas MD Anderson Cancer Center, Clinical Professor of Pediatrics at the University of Southern California, and Adjunct Professor of Biological Sciences at California Polytechnic State University, San Luis Obispo, where he lives. Married with 10 children and 16 grandchildren, he had an important role in the critical early years of leukaemia treatment research at Roswell Park Cancer Center in Buffalo. He was also the Founding Director of the outstanding St Jude Childrens' Research Hospital in Memphis. His productive efforts to initiate curative therapy of childhood acute leukaemia and to develop coordinated combination treatment of all childhood cancers have been recognised by many national and international awards. Despite his considerable work as a researcher, teacher and administrator, he has always managed to continue his primary perspective as a caring childrens' doctor.

He has witnessed and contributed vitally to the transition of childhood leukaemia from a fatal to a curable condition.

A Scientist

Mel Greaves is Professor of Cell Biology and Chairman of the Section of Haemato-Oncology at the Institute of Cancer Research and Royal Marsden Hospital in London. Married with two children, Mel has spent thirty years investigating the biology of childhood leukaemia. His research has provided new diagnostic screens and has led to an understanding of the cellular origins of leukaemia. His research has also provided insight to its molecular lesions and their timing, before birth, as well as the possible causes of the disease. Mel's research has been recognised by many distinguished international awards and prizes and also by his election to The Royal Society. Professor Greaves has published more than 400 research papers. He is the co-editor of a major textbook on leukaemia and the author of a popular science book *"Cancer. The Evolutionary Legacy"*. He strongly supports the measures to improve the public understanding of science.

> *He has witnessed the transition of leukaemia from a biomedical mystery to an illness that is understood and more effectively controlled.*

A Family

Janine Louise Fernandes is 17 and an outstanding student at Newstead Wood School for Girls in Orpington, Kent (one of the top selective schools in the UK). She was diagnosed with acute lymphoblastic leukaemia at the age 4 years old. After two years of successful chemotherapy treatment and a lot of support from the doctors and her family, she is now in long term remission. She is optimistic for her future and has a zest for life. She has also lectured to her school chums on leukaemia.

> *Janine has witnessed childhood leukaemia — very first hand.*

Delena Fernandes is Janine's mum. She was born in Nairobi, Kenya in April 1964. She immigrated to London in 1970 where she continued her schooling. She now works for the local government as a Childcare Development Officer. She took a career break to take care of Janine during her illness. Along with her husband, she has drawn strengths from her daughter's ordeals.

> *She has witnessed a child, her child, with leukaemia, first hand.*

A Mother

Nicola Horlick was born in Nottingham in 1960. After attending Cheltenham Ladies' College and Birkenhead High School GDST, she became one of the first female undergraduates at Balliol College, Oxford, where she read Jurisprudence. Nicola then enjoyed a glittering career as a businesswoman and fund manager with leading companies. At the same time, Nicola married and had six children. One of them, Georgina, was diagnosed with leukaemia in 1989. After two relapses and a bone marrow transplant, Georgina sadly died. Georgina's illness prompted Nicola to get involved in a number of leukaemia, cancer and children's charities. In 1997, she wrote a book entitled *"Can You Have It All?"* with all the proceeds going to Great Ormond Street Hospital.

She has also witnessed a child, her child, with leukaemia, first hand.

A Paediatric Psychologist

Dr Jeanette EWM van Dongen-Melman is a clinical child psychologist, psychotherapist and behaviour therapist at the Department of Clinical Psychology at Ikazia Hospital in Rotterdam, the Netherlands. She started her research on the long-term psychosocial consequences of childhood cancer in 1982 at the Erasmus Medical Center-Sophia Children's Hospital in Rotterdam. She investigated the impact of long-term psychosocial consequences on the former cancer patients as well as on their parents and siblings. Analysing formatted answers from existing questionnaires, she wanted her research to convey the entire family's experiences and perspectives. She aimed for an approach in which interviews with the child, parents and siblings, along with observations in their homes, were combined with newly developed illness-specific questionnaires and existing clinical questionnaires. The results of this approach were described in her PhD thesis *"On surviving childhood cancer"*. She has published more than 50 papers, including two patients' booklets, of which one has been translated into six languages. Dr van Dongen-Melman strongly advocates the use of clinical psychological methods in the medical treatment of chronically ill children, in particular those with cancer. This is because the illness and treatment, on top of the additional pressure on the normal development of children, affects their quality of life. To decrease the stresses inherent in the illness experience, Dr van Dongen-Melman developed a behavioural therapy training program for the parents of children with leukaemia to reduce the behavioural side effects of medications, in particular corticosteroids. She is married to Professor Jacques JM van Dongen MD, who is an international researcher in childhood leukaemia.

> *She has witnessed the many psychological difficulties faced by children with leukaemia and their families.*

THE ARTIST'S BIOSKETCH

The Artist: Susan Macfarlane

Susan Macfarlane was born in Sussex in 1938. After training at the Winchester School of Art under David Peare, her longing to travel took her to the Far East. In 1963, she moved to Greece, where she studied for a year under the painter John Dragoumis. After marriage in 1964, Susan moved to France where her two sons were born. While raising her family, she continued to paint with this period of work showing the stark and romantic hills of her home in the Basses Alpes — massive rock shapes in space, upon which man has made so little impression. During this time, a commission to design stained glass for the Anglican church in Cannes led to an absorbing period of studying the ancient technique with the master glazier, Alan Peinado.

After returning to England in 1986, Susan's choice of subject changed dramatically. Drawing the prehistoric sites of Wiltshire and watching the modern visitors and their reactions, she developed an intense sense of human continuity and endeavour. She built on this sense by observing people at work, their machinery and their instruments. Susan drew her subjects from life, which required intense concentration and powers of observation, later producing the paintings in her studio from her studies.

Following the success of the widely toured exhibition of *A Picture of Health* — paintings and drawings on breast cancer care — Susan spent two years continuing to link art and medicine. Working in close collaboration with Dr Geoffrey Farrer-Brown, she sketched and then painted scenes of childhood leukaemia. She had followed the lives of children and their parents, in London, Bristol, Gloucester and Manchester, thus experiencing the very demanding treatment required to defeat leukaemia. The resultant collection of 27 oil paintings and drawings entitled _Living with Leukaemia_ are curated by Dr Farrer-Brown and have been publicly exhibited.

One Man Shows in the UK include:-
Patricia Wells Gallery, Bristol, 1979
British Council Exhibition, Brussels, 1980
Archaeological Museum Gallery, Devizes, 1982, _"Ancient Wiltshire"_
Arts Council Affiliated Exhibition, Leicester, 1985
The Subscription Rooms, Stroud, 1992, _"The Woollen Mills of Stroud — An artist's impression"_
Archaeological Museum Gallery, Devizes, 1993, _"An Artist in Ancient Gozo"_
The Foyer Gallery, Barbican Centre, London, 1995, _"A Picture of Health"_
This exhibition then toured to Edinburgh, Nottingham, Cardiff, Manchester, Oxford, Birmingham and Bristol.
Brown's Gallery, Tain, Ross-shire, 1996, _"Balblair — A working distillery"_
The Foyer Gallery, Barbican Centre, London, 1998, _"Living with Leukaemia"_, a touring exhibition

The Institute of Child Health, London, April/May 2008, _"Living with Leukaemia"_.

In 1998, Susan Macfarlane was one of 48 living artists commissioned to design and paint a stamp to mark the millennium. The event was described by the Royal Mail as "the largest and most prestigious commissioning by the Royal Mail". The stamp painted by Susan was entitled "Nursing Care" and was one of four stamps for the month of

March 1999 which recorded "The Patient's Tale". The theme of her stamp was chosen to commemorate the work of Florence Nightingale in raising the status of nursing to that of a caring profession.

Susan tragically died following an accident at her home in Petersfield, Hampshire on 14th August 2002.

Donald Pinkel

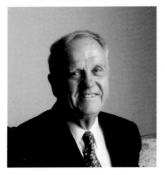

Susan MacFarlane

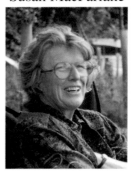

Mel Greaves

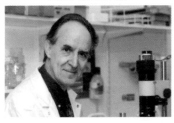

Nicola Horlick

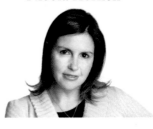

Jeanette van Dongen-Melman

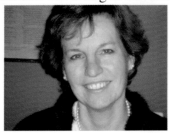

Delena Fernandes

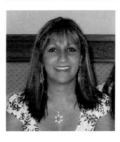

Janine Fernandes

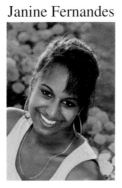

INTRODUCTION TO CHILDHOOD LEUKAEMIA

Mel Greaves and Donald Pinkel

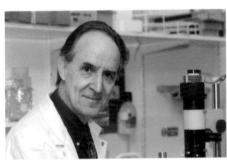
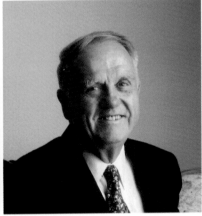

INTRODUCTION TO CHILDHOOD LEUKAEMIA

Mel Greaves and Donald Pinkel

Leukaemia is a cancer of blood cells, as are lymphoma and myeloma. In common with all cancers, they are cellular disorders driven by mutations or modifications of DNA, our genetic code. In an individual patient with leukaemia all the leukaemic cells are a clone; the progeny of a single, disordered blood cell.

Leukaemia accounts for a modest fraction of adult cancers ($\sim 7\%$) and, although substantially rarer (by 10 fold) in children, leukaemia is the major type of paediatric cancer, accounting for around one third of all cases. Cancer occurs throughout the animal kingdom. Several mammalian species, especially domesticated cats, cattle and chickens develop leukaemia. Medical records from antiquity in Greece and India backtrack the presence of cancers from more than 2000 years ago. In that sense, cancer is not a modern disease, as often asserted. But some cancers are easier to detect than others e.g. those of the breast and skin for example. Leukaemia posed a problem in this respect. It may well have existed at some level throughout human history but in the absence of microscopy, this "liquid" cancer would have escaped detection. Patients with leukaemia then would have died of infection or haemorrhage without a diagnosis. It was therefore not until the mid-19th century (with the emergence of microscopy and cellular pathology) that leukaemia was first observed.

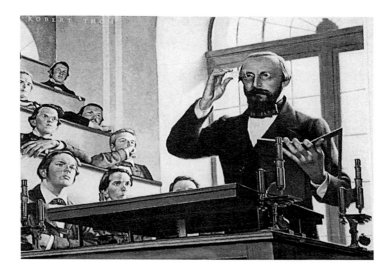

Fig. 1.   Rudolf Virchow, German cellular pathologist.

In 1845, a young medical doctor, Rudolf Virchow (Fig. 1), observed a patient with complaints of weakness and pallor. The patient had a large spleen and her blood was near white because of very few red blood cells and excessive white blood cells. He reported this case in a medical journal classifying it as a case of "white blood". He thought it was a new disease. His seniors doubted this idea; they considered this patient a victim of infectious disease. The high white blood cell levels were a reaction to infection. This opinion was similar when a French and two contemporary Scottish physicians published similar case reports.

But unlike the others, young Dr Virchow embarked on an intensive investigation of his "new" disease. He gathered more cases of this fatal disorder and studied their gross and microscopic anatomical findings as well as clinical features. A decade later he published a detailed monograph including meticulous hand drawings of what he now called "leukaemia", Greek for white blood. From these observations, he postulated the cellular theory of leukaemia. The disease was caused by uncontrolled replication of a disordered blood cell precursor with growth and survival advantages over normal blood cell precursors. This unregulated proliferation eventually interfered with normal body function, resulting in the death of the patient. Virchow's theory remains essentially correct 150 years later. It was elaborated by newer discoveries in cell and molecular biology and genetics as highlighted elsewhere in this book.

Most of the cases of leukaemia described by Rudolph Virchow and other European pathologists in the mid-19th century were adults. From their brief descriptions and rather superficial microscopic evidence, it was probable that most of these patients were suffering from chronic myeloid leukaemias. A more detailed classification of leukaemia awaited the discoveries of Paul Ehrlich in the 1880s. Ehrlich discovered aniline dyes that could stain blood films which distinguish the morphology of different types of myeloid and lymphoid blood cells. Ehrlich, and later the Swiss haematologist Naegeli, had the insight that clinically acute leukaemia involved "primitive" cells from the bone marrow that developed into distinctive myeloid and lymphoid lineages (Fig. 2). Thus was coined the terms acute lymphoblastic leukaemia (ALL) and acute myeloblastic leukaemia (AML). Anecdotal reports of leukaemia in children appeared in the late 19th century. By the turn of the century (1904), Churchill, a physician in Chicago, had described a series of children (15 cases) diagnosed with ALL. Their duration of disease before death was short (a few days to a few months) and the age range was newborn to 10 years.

The classification of acute leukaemia in children and adults are usually two major varieties, ALL and AML. This remained grounded in the simple morphology of the dye-stained cells until the 1970s, when immunologists introduced antibodies that could reliably distinguish different types of morphologically anonymous lymphoid cells. Consequently, ALL was subdivided into subsets corresponding to B lineage precursors and T lineage precursors. In the 1980s, scientists carried out subcellular dissection of leukaemic cell diversity at the level of chromosome structure and then at the level of DNA. They discovered the critical and diverse underlying molecular patholology

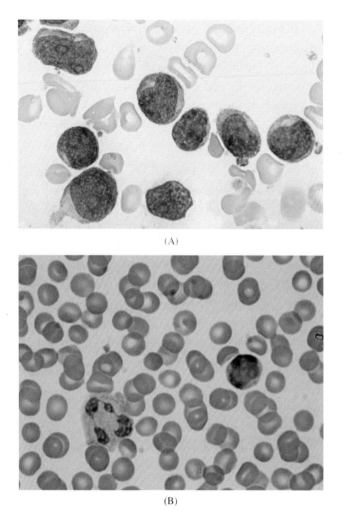

Fig. 2.   Leukaemic (ALL) (A) versus normal blood (B). Courtesy of Dr B Bain. (A) The
nucleus of the leukaemic cells is stained red by special dyes. (B) Two normal white cells in
sea of smaller red cells. Large cell lower left is granulocyte. Round cell at 3.o'clock with
purple stained nucleus is normal lymphocyte.

that drives the diseases. The classification that emerges from these
sequential insights over the decades is a branching tree-like structure
(Fig. 3) used in the haematology laboratories of many hospitals.

Modern human genome scanning methods indicate that each
patient's leukaemic cells have followed a unique evolutionary tra-
jectory as a novel subspecies of cell. The consequence is that each

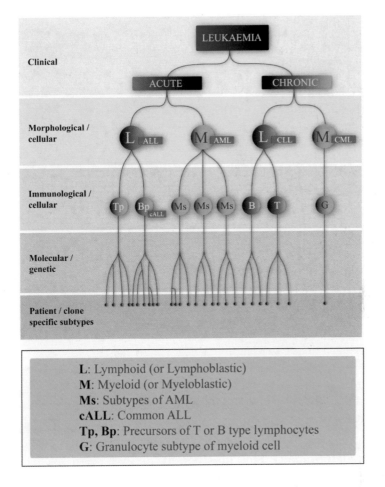

Fig. 3.   Hierarchical classification of leukaemia.

patient's leukaemia ends up represented by an individual leaf on a specific twig or a particular branch of the tree. The prevalence of the major branching subtypes of childhood leukaemia vary according to age. The peak incidence of disease at ages two to five years old reflects mostly the "common" or B cell precursor variant of ALL (Fig. 4).

Most cancers probably harbour a similar degree of complexity which, in part at least, may explain some of their general intransigence to successful therapy — they are not *one* disease. The degree

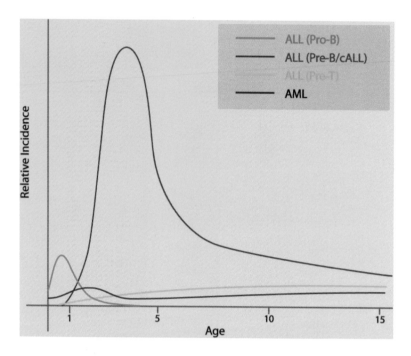

Fig. 4.   Age distribution of main subtypes of childhood leukaemia.

of cellular, chromosomal and molecular diversity in leukaemia raises some difficult but important practical issues and opportunities. At what level of cellular and molecular characteristics is response to therapy determined? This must surely depend upon the particular therapy itself which has been continually modified and tailored to cellular subtype. Currently in leukaemia, and cancer in general, it appears that abnormal genotype, i.e. altered chromosomes and genes, has a major impact on clinical response and outcome. This can be rationalised as we now know that the altered or mutated genome influences the signal pathways in cells that control life or death of those cells in the face of therapeutic drugs or irradiation. The patterns of distinctive genetic change in leukaemic cells also provide potentially ideal therapeutic targets since they uniquely distinguish leukaemic from normal cells. But, this in turn poses a very considerable dilemma for cancer and leukaemia therapeutics. Do we design and tailor novel therapeutics to match each patient — with all the technical and major financial implications this would entail — or do we continue to strive to identify shared, generic features of leukaemia that provide common therapeutic targets? Currently, both avenues are being explored very actively.

Childhood acute leukaemia occurs throughout the world, though it appears that the incidence rate of ALL is significantly higher (perhaps by 10 fold) in more affluent or developed countries. In the latter, the annual incidence rate is at around 30 to 40 cases per one million children which, for paediatric populations in the UK or the USA, translates to around 450 or 2,750 new cases each year respectively. In absolute terms, the risk of any child developing acute leukaemia between birth and age 15 years (in Europe, Australia or the USA) is approximately one in 2000.

The initial, clinical diagnosis of childhood leukaemia relates to the pathology, the common symptoms being paleness (anaemia), bleeding tendency, fatigue, aches and pains and unexplained fevers. Collectively, they reflect the highjack of normal bone marrow function by leukaemic cells. Treatment, as described in the chapter by Donald Pinkel, is now relatively complex and consists of chemotherapy with several drugs in different combinations and various schedules for approximately 3 years. In the case of Janine (Chapter 6), this was effective and curative. When standard chemotherapy fails, intensive chemotherapy using drugs and/or drug schedules not included in the initial treatment can be curative in many children.

Very high dose chemotherapy followed by haematopoietic stem cell transplant to replenish the child's blood cell system with donor graft cells (and produce an immune reaction to the leukaemia) has been used for over three decades. This procedure can be curative but is associated with a relatively high procedure-related early death rate and long term disability and late death. This negative outcome is largely due to reaction of the donor immune system to the child's normal organs and tissues but also to side effects of the drugs used to suppress the reaction. This was the case, sadly, for Georgie whose story is told in Chapter 5. Meaningful comparisons of haematopoietic stem cell transplant methods versus intent to cure "salvage chemotherapy" for children with relapsed ALL have been conducted in the United Kingdom and the United States. They demonstrate no advantage in cure or quality of survival for transplant methods.

Despite the success in treating childhood leukaemia (cure rates are reported to be 80%) for some children with ALL, much remains to be done. Closer attention is needed to monitoring the effects of each element of treatment on growth and development of the children to healthy, happy, fulfilled adults. The eventual risk/benefit ratio of each element must be weighed and reweighed in deciding on current treatment.

The challenges for the future lie in the development of more specific biologically targeted treatment and in preventive measures derived from the understanding of the causes and mechanisms of leukaemia. Perhaps then, the many children worldwide currently without access to curative treatment will be reached.

A PAEDIATRICIAN'S JOURNEY

Donald Pinkel

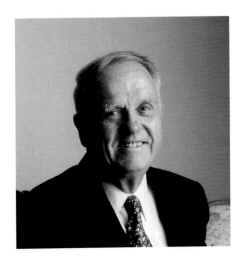

A PAEDIATRICIAN'S JOURNEY

Donald Pinkel

My journey with children with leukaemia and their families began in 1949. The diagnosis of acute leukaemia then was a death warrant and few survived other types of childhood cancer. Since I became committed to my fellow travellers in 1953, research and treatment of children with leukaemia and other forms of cancer has been the main thread of my career. I have had the privilege of working with them and their families and with many other physicians and scientists to understand their diseases and develop curative treatments. We have been assisted by numerous skilled nurses, pharmacists, technologists, social workers and nurses' aides. We have been supported by government and private funding agencies as well as countless volunteers who donate blood, raise money and help out parents. All working together have radically changed the outlook for children with cancer. Approximately 75–80% of children with the most frequent form, acute lymphoblastic leukaemia, can now be cured. Estimated 5 year survival of all childhood cancers in developed countries is over 70%. However, there is much more to be done!

The characteristic leukaemia of children is acute lymphoblastic leukaemia (ALL). This chapter focuses on ALL because it best illustrates progress in curing leukaemia. It is also used widely as a model in understanding how cancer develops.

Childhood ALL usually affects healthy, well cared for children, most frequently between two and five years old, but often during early infancy or adolescence, also. They tend to become mysteriously ill over weeks or months with unexplained fevers, loss of appetite, fatigue, reduced activity, headaches, pains in joints and abdomen, and sometimes changes in personality. Easy bruising and nosebleeds signify bleeding disorder and pallor, anaemia. Sometimes swollen lymph nodes in the neck persist and enlarge after a nose and throat infection subsides. Childhood ALL is a great imitator capable of mimicking any childhood disease including rheumatic fever, kidney and liver disorders, bowel obstruction, meningitis, and even brain tumours.

Initial examination may be apparently normal, prompting repeat visits. But eventually pallor, fever, large lymph nodes, spleen and liver, pinpoint skin haemorrhages called petechiae, and extensive bruises prompt complete clinical investigations for diagnosis. The results can be variable but, low haemoglobin and red blood cell levels, low platelet counts, and abnormal white blood cells are characteristic. The white blood cell count itself can be low or high. The examination of a stained smear of bone marrow aspirated by a needle from the hip or spine bones usually confirms the diagnosis of ALL (Fig. 2). The clinical features of ALL are caused by the occupation of blood-forming tissues in the bone marrow, spleen and lymph nodes by an abnormal rapidly growing clone of lymphoblasts. These cells also infiltrate most organs and tissues of the body.

The course of untreated childhood ALL is brief, averaging about six weeks. Death is due to anaemia, bleeding, infection, or inter-ference with a vital organ function by leukaemic infiltration.

Types of Childhood ALL

As outlined in the introductory chapter, there are biologically different subtypes of ALL. The distinction between them is important because they present different problems and require different treatment plans. Also important in treatment planning are the chromosomal and gene characteristics of childhood ALL. For example, children whose ALL demonstrates excessive numbers of chromosomes usually have a high cure rate without the need for more risky treatments. Those with an abnormally small chromosome number 22, called the Philadelphia chromosome, and resulting from a reciprocal translocation (= exchange of chunks of DNA or large chromosomal regions) between chromosomes 9 and 22, usually need more risky treatment.

Early Treatment of Childhood ALL

In the 19th and early 20th centuries, there is little mention of childhood leukaemia or of attempts to modify its fatal course in medical literature. In 1865, arsenious trioxide, used for syphilis, was shown to produce temporary relief and the reduction of white blood cells in chronic leukaemia of adults. Radiation therapy, introduced at the beginning of the 20th century, produced similar effects. The first report of cure appeared in 1930. A Swiss physician gave a young adult with myelocytic leukaemia arsenious trioxide, mesothorium, radiation therapy, and blood transfusions from two siblings. After a difficult recovery, he remained free of leukaemia for the rest of his long life.

When I was a medical student, childhood ALL was uniformly fatal. When the diagnosis was suspected, a consultant haematologist or pathologist was summoned to aspirate bone marrow and examine stained smears of blood and marrow. The diagnosis was confirmed and conveyed to the child's physician, who had the task of informing the parents of the grim prognosis. Blood transfusions, analgesics, and possibly an antibacterial drug were given to delay death, while the family tried to adjust to the loss of their child. There was little or no counselling and the parents often felt isolated because of the fear and silence surrounding the disease. These attitudes were very much the same as those encountered when children began developing acquired human immunodeficiency disease (AIDS) three decades later.

In the teaching hospitals, there were similar attitudes. When on morning ward rounds we came to a child with leukaemia, the word was whispered, everyone looked glum and we moved on to the next patient. When parents were present, they felt abandoned. Some felt they were being punished for some imaginary fault. For religious families, clergy were comforting with messages of "God's will" and "their own little angel in heaven."

Many nurses, true to their profession, worked closely with the children and their parents to help them understand leukaemia. They provided comfort and caring but also reminded physicians to address the childrens' needs for supportive measures such as analgesia and the parents' needs to talk with them.

In June 1948, as I completed my first year of medical school at the University of Buffalo, a light appeared for children with ALL. Professor Sidney Farber (Fig. 5) and colleagues in Boston reported that

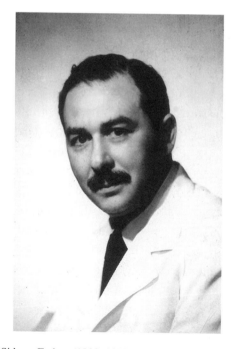

Fig. 5. Professor Sidney Farber (1903–1973) and colleagues at Lederle Laboratories developed the anti-folate compounds aminopterin and methotrexate, the first drugs to produce remissions in children with acute lymphoblastic leukaemia (ALL). This began the road to cure.

a new synthetic chemical compound, 4-amino pteroylglutamic acid or aminopterin, produced complete remissions in some children with ALL. Farber had noticed a resemblance between the lymphoblasts of ALL and the erythroblasts of megaloblastic anaemia of infancy, a disease cured by the vitamin, pteroylglutamic acid, also called folic acid. However, when he gave folic acid to children with ALL, their leukaemia seemed to accelerate instead. On his advice, colleagues at Lederle's laboratories then developed aminopterin as an antagonist of folic acid by adding the 4-amino group.

The complete remissions described by Farber and colleagues consisted of the complete disappearance of leukaemia cells in the blood and bone marrow (Fig. 2), the return of blood cell counts to normal, the relief of all symptoms and normal physical examinations. However, the remissions were temporary and leukaemia resistant to aminopterin recurred within months despite its continued administration. Aminopterin also produced folic acid deficiency in normal tissues with resultant pathology and clinical disorders; this seriously limited dosage. However, the light of hope for eventual cure of ALL by drugs was lit and many scientists responded with new research to develop treatment for ALL.

In the winter of 1949, I elected to study haematology with Professor David Miller at the county hospital. I was given a vial of aminopterin and sent to the laboratory to find if I could block the toxic effects of aminopterin in rats with cobalt. Unfortunately, the cobalt was more toxic than the aminopterin. I learned how to handle failure. However, I also learned how to interpret bone marrow preparations provided by Dr Miller and examined patients with him and his staff. There I saw my first child with ALL and felt the heartbreak. At that time, both my mentor and other haematologists were reluctant to use aminopterin or its derivative methotrexate because of their toxic effects.

Upon graduation in 1951, I started residency in paediatrics at the Children's Hospital of Buffalo. I soon found that childhood ALL and other forms of cancer were among the leading causes of death there. Our haematologist was part time and we had no oncologist, so I was readily drawn to look after children with ALL and other cancers. We now had two other drugs, besides the antifolates aminopterin and methotrexate that produced temporary complete remissions of ALL.

In 1950, the recently isolated and synthesized cortisone, a hormone derived from the adrenal gland, was found to cause regression of ALL. This allows the regeneration of normal bone marrow and blood cells. The remissions were usually brief and accompanied by serious metabolic disorders such as high blood sugar, increased fatty acids, protein wastage, potassium depletion, and a peculiar obesity. Later, we discovered that its action against ALL was linked to the acceleration of natural cell death of lymphocytes and lymphoblasts.

In 1951, Drs Joseph Burchenal, David Karnofsky and others produced complete remissions of childhood ALL with mercaptopurine. This synthetic drug was the result of years of brilliant research by George Hitchings and Gertrude Elion in the Burroughs Wellcome laboratories (Fig. 6A). Using the new knowledge of deoxyribonucleic acid (DNA) chemistry, they searched for the derivatives of the purine bases that are at the heart of DNA. Their aim was to exploit the potential differences in DNA metabolism between normal and cancer cells in order to develop chemical compounds specifically effective in destroying cancer cells. Mercaptopurine, an analog of the essential purine base guanine becomes modified and incorporated into DNA synthesis in place of guanine. Once incorporated into the DNA synthesis of lymphoblasts, it serves as a poison that interferes with further DNA synthesis, and therefore further replication of the lymphoblasts. As with aminopterin and methotrexate, its effects are not so specific and normal cells and tissues are also affected. Again, dosage is limited by toxicity. Mercaptopurine is the first antileukaemia drug to be designed and synthesized specifically for this purpose rather than the result of a chance observation.

Hitchings and Elion designed and synthesized two other life saving drugs used in children with leukaemia. Acycloguanosine (acyclovir) cures potentially fatal herpes and chickenpox infections.

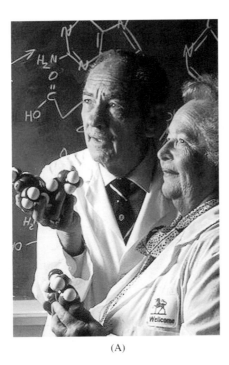

(A)

Fig. 6A.   George Hitchings (1905–1998) and Gertrude Elion (1918–1999) used new understanding of molecular biology to synthesize drugs targeted at DNA replication. One of them, mercaptopurine, was the second drug to produce lasting remissions in children with ALL. The combination of methotrexate and mercaptopurine remains the most valuable treatement more than half a century later. These scientists are also responsible for two life saving drugs used for complications of ALL.

Allopurinol prevents one of the dangerous complications of sudden destruction of ALL cells by chemotherapy.

Following the lead of Drs Farber and Burchenal, in Buffalo we used the combination of cortisone and oral daily methotrexate to induce remission and then methotrexate alone to maintain remission until the inevitable relapse with methotrexate-resistant ALL. For children whose ALL relapsed or did not respond initially, we gave the combination of cortisone and oral daily mercaptopurine to induce remission and then mercaptopurine alone to maintain it until again drug resistance led to relapse and eventual death. With this simple plan and supportive measures like blood transfusion and antibiotics, the majority of children experienced remissions and survived with good health and activity for many months, sometimes more than a year. But the tragedy of childhood death was delayed, not overcome. For us, as well as for the families, we felt that we were so close but yet so far from curing the children.

As chief resident in 1953 to 1954, I decided to devote my career to children with leukaemia and other forms of cancer. With a small grant from the local cancer society I established a childhood cancer and leukaemia service, clinic and registry in the Children's Hospital and began monthly multi-specialty tumour boards. All agreed this was appropriate but many felt it was futile: "Childhood cancer is hopeless until we know its cause and besides cancer is an adult not a paediatric problem." "Don't give those poisons; let the children die in peace." "Don't waste your career pursuing a hopeless cause." However, I had developed an emotional attachment to the children with cancer and their families. I was especially concerned with the sense of isolation and abandonment they experienced. The least one might accomplish is to give them the reassurance that they were cared for and cared about by personal attention and by vigorous search for new understanding of their diseases and investigation of new ways to treat them. I felt a personal obligation because I was more familiar than others with the children, their families and their suffering.

Working with Professor Sidney Farber

In 1955, after military service that left me partially paraplegic from paralytic poliomyelitis, I met Professor Sidney Farber at the Boston Children's Hospital Medical Center. He was the head of pathology and the director of the Children's Cancer Research Foundation and its clinical services, the Jimmy Fund Clinic. This was the Mecca of childhood cancer research and treatment. Generously, he put me to work while I continued outpatient rehabilitation at a veterans' hospital. Besides caring for children in the clinic, I was assigned to evaluate a new chemical compound in children whose leukaemia or other fatal cancers were resistant to known treatments. The compound was Actinomycin D, an antibiotic isolated from a soil bacillus by Dr Waksman at Rutgers University. It was anti-leukaemic in experimental mice.

Actinomycin D was given to children with ALL resistant to mercaptopurine and methotrexate and to others with cancers for which there was no available effective treatment. In leukaemia, it reduced the abnormal blood cell levels and leukaemic organ size but there was no regeneration of normal bone marrow or blood cell counts. Toxicity was serious. However, it did have some dramatic effects in destroying embryonal rhabdomyosarcoma, a soft tissue cancer in children, and Wilm's tumour, the kidney cancer of children. This was the first drug to affect these cancers and the first natural antibiotic shown to be effective in human cancer.

We began to use actinomycin D after the surgical removal of Wilm's tumour or rhabdomyosarcoma to prevent development of spread to the lungs, which is a frequent event. This was the beginning of adjuvant chemotherapy, a common practice now in the treatment of many types of cancer with a variety of drugs. We also used actinomycin D to shrink large unresectable cancers of these two types in order to allow surgical removal and avoid highly radical surgery or to permit more conservative radiation therapy. This was the beginning of neo adjuvant chemotherapy, also used widely now for many cancers with other drugs as well as actinomycin.

Some time later, it was discovered that actinomycin inhibited the transcription of ribonucleic acid (RNA) from DNA. It became an important tool in virus research, and led to the discovery of reverse transcriptase, used now for DNA identification. It also led to the recognition of the retroviruses such as human immunodeficiency virus (HIV), associated with AIDS, and human T-cell leukaemia virus (HTLV-1), a cause of an unusual type of adult leukaemia/lymphoma.

Dr Farber and his clinic director, Dr Rudy Toch, directed the treatment of each new patient. They were resistant to the use of standardised, written treatment protocols, pointing out that each child was different and each ALL or other cancer was different. Therefore, drug dosage, combination and sequence must be individualised and integrated into the child's total treatment and comprehensive medical and psychosocial services. Dr Farber called this concept "total care." While I appreciated the need for customising care to the person, I thought it necessary to establish well designed and conscientiously followed written protocols in order to ask key questions and obtain reliable answers. Scientifically valid new information is essential to progress.

As valuable my experience, as generous was Dr Farber, and as well the children were being treated, I needed to move on to a more scientific research approach to childhood ALL. However, Dr Farber's admonition, "to terminate or alter any course of treatment if the continued survival or comfort of the patient requires it", found its place later when we inserted a clause to this effect in all our research treatment protocols. His concept of "total care" of the child with cancer is practiced almost without exception in children's cancer services today.

As with other children's cancer services, the policy in Boston was to conceal the diagnosis of cancer from the patients and to obfuscate when they asked questions. I had an epiphany one day when a 14 year old boy I was examining asked me if he were going to die soon. When I inquired why he was asking this question he said that his friends had told him that he had leukaemia and that he would die of it. He went on to say that he did not believe his friends because he trusted his parents and his doctors and knew they would tell him something so important; they would not lie to him. I felt a knife in my heart. I was a traitor to my patient. I resolved then to always tell the diagnosis to children regardless of age.

Paediatrics at Roswell Park Cancer Center

In 1956, I was appointed the first paediatrician at Roswell Park Cancer Centre in Buffalo. My charge was to initiate a childhood cancer research and treatment department. I joined Jim Holland who was the head of the adult leukaemia department, Tom Frei and Jay Freireich of the National Cancer Institute, and others to conduct multi-institutional collaborative studies of acute leukaemia treatment. We inaugurated some of the first written protocol studies designed to scientifically compare various regimens of ALL therapy, including combinations of methotrexate and mercaptopurine that resulted in longer remissions and survival in many patients. We also tested new agents in patients with ALL resistant to the available effective drugs.

Among the new agents was cyclophosphamide, a synthetic compound developed in Germany. Its story harks back to World War I when sulphur mustard gas victims suffered severe bone marrow damage and low white blood cell counts and to the Bari, Italy disaster in World War II when the townspeople developed similar effects when a ship in port carrying the gas exploded. The study of the Bari disaster led to the idea that a solid form of the gas might be an antileukaemic agent. Nitrogen mustard, also called mechlorethamine, was synthesized and found effective in lymph node cancers, including Hodgkin's disease, for which it is still used. In ALL, the drug reduced leukaemia mass but was very toxic and did not produce remissions.

Linking the mechlorethamine chemically to a ring compound resulted in cyclophosphamide, which was more stable than the parent compound, and easier to administer. It also had independent activity against ALL. It became a component of some treatment plans for childhood ALL in 1959.

Another drug became available for childhood ALL in 1961. The search for new anti-diabetes drugs at Eli Lilly laboratories and the University of Western Ontario yielded chemical compounds from the periwinkle plant that lowered white blood cell counts in mice with leukaemia. Clinical evaluation in children showed that one of the compounds, vincristine, produced complete remissions of ALL in children with leukaemia resistant to the other anti-leukaemia drugs. It acts by binding to tubulin, a prime constituent of microtubules essential to cell division, cell skeleton and cell motility, and of nerve fibres. Vincristine induced remissions quickly and did not interfere with the resurgence of normal blood cell formation. However, the remissions tended to be short and nerve damage serious, especially with prolonged or frequent exposure.

While at Roswell Park, I studied the epidemiology of childhood ALL in the area, finding a socioeconomic relationship and residential aggregation that might be consistent with a viral causation. I also set up a virus laboratory to search for a childhood leukaemia virus, a search which continued in my next position.

The relatively small, compact paediatric unit at Roswell Park provided opportunities to form a team, a "therapeutic community" of parents, children and staff to work together in attempts to reduce fear and suffering while providing the best available care and conducting relevant research. Hospitalisation was minimised, around the clock visiting and "rooming-in" allowed, local housing used for patients and family members from distant places; and analgesic administration optimised. All patient care and drugs were free at Roswell Park. This was an important attribute that still remains a necessity to assure the opportunity of all children to be cured of cancer.

St Jude Children's Research Hospital

In 1961, I was appointed the first director of St Jude Children's Research Hospital in Memphis, Tennessee, founded by entertainer Danny Thomas (Fig. 6B) with the support of friends in Hollywood and Memphis and Americans of Lebanese and Syrian descent. The construction was completed, a core medical, basic science, nursing and administrative staff was recruited and the hospital opened in 1962.

Among the founding precepts was complete racial integration at all levels and in all ways, a radical notion in the Mid-South and Mississippi Delta area, if not in the entire United States. Another was the provision of completely free services to all children accepted for study and care including transportation, local room and board, medication and, when needed, food and clothing, in order to further assure accessibility. Federal agencies, especially the National Cancer Institute,

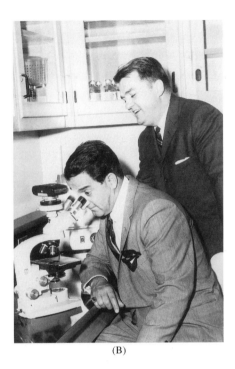

(B)

Fig. 6B.   Danny Thomas and Donald Pinkel. Entertainer Danny Thomas (1914–1991), Founder (sitting), and Donald Pinkel, Founding Director (standing), at the dedication of St Jude Children's Research Hospital, February 1962.

helped finance the construction and infrastructure and, within a short while, much of the basic and clinical research. An affiliation with the University of Tennessee provided academic appointments, students and paediatric residents. It also helped to recruit research and clinical fellows.

One of the programs initiated was the search for a cure for childhood ALL. Despite the development of six effective drugs for ALL in the past years, "cure" was still a forbidden word because of the pessimism that prevailed about the possibility of curing generalised cancer as well as the experience that drug treatment had only prolonged survival, not cured. "Hopeless" was still the concept and "Let them die in peace" remained a practice among many physicians.

Based on clinical observations of the previous decade, my colleagues at St Jude and I (Fig. 7) identified four major obstacles to

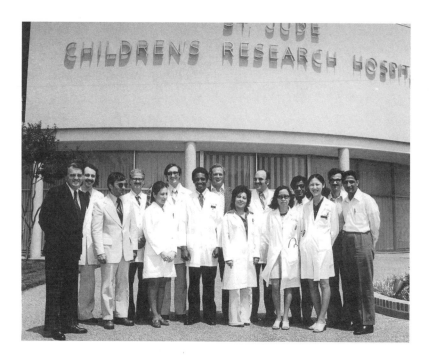

Fig. 7.   Clinical research staff at St Jude Children's Research Hospital (1969).

cure of childhood ALL in 1962. First was drug resistance, initial or acquired. In many instances, ALL did not respond to a drug and, in others, initially responsive ALL relapsed and progressed despite its continued administration. Secondly, the toxic effects were often over-lapping, especially with regard to the depression of immune response, the destruction of normal blood forming cells, and the damage to mucous membranes. This overlapping toxicity limited the dosage of drug combinations and risked a drug being given in insufficient dose to be effective. Insufficient dosage over time encourages drug resistance.

Third was leukaemic relapse in the central nervous system, specif-ically in the soft covering that surrounds the brain and spinal cord and their arteries and veins. This soft covering is called the leptomeninges. Within its two layers is a clear salty fluid, the cerebrospinal fluid, which circulates in the leptomeninges around the brain and spinal cord and their arteries and veins. The relapse tends to occur during otherwise complete remission of ALL. The early symptoms are those of meningitis: stiff neck, headache, vomiting and leukaemia cells in the cerebrospinal fluid. Symptoms can become more grievous with brain damage, convulsions and paralyses when the leptomeningeal leukaemia invades the brain itself or leukaemic masses around the arteries choke off circulation of blood to the brain.

The reason for leukaemic relapse during chemotherapy is the failure of the more effective drugs, methotrexate and mercaptopurine, as well as less effective drugs like vincristine to penetrate into the cerebrospinal fluid. Since ALL is a systemic disease, the ALL cells are usually present in the leptomeninges at diagnosis. When not reached by sufficient drug these cells are free to replicate while the same cells elsewhere are being destroyed. This results in leptomeningeal relapse while the child is otherwise in complete remission. I had encountered leptomeningeal relapse in children when in Boston and at Roswell Park. It was treated by direct injection of methotrexate into the spinal fluid or by modest doses of cranial radiation therapy with temporary relief. By 1962, with longer survival of children with ALL due to drug treatment, almost 50% of children experienced initial relapse in the leptomeninges and eventually the brain itself.

Perhaps the fourth obstacle was the most formidable: pessimism. The conventional wisdom that ALL is incurable was a self-imposed imprisonment of imagination and almost a self-fulfilling prophecy.

"Total Therapy" of ALL

Based on all we knew from clinical experience, cooperative trials, mouse leukaemia experiments, cell culture studies and the new molecular biology, we devised a strategy of childhood ALL treatment that we called "Total Therapy" shortly after the hospital's opening. It consisted of four phases.

The first phase is induction of complete remission. The purpose is to reduce the mass of ALL to allow the regeneration of normal blood forming cells and thus normal blood cell counts, their return to normal activity, and relief from symptoms and signs of disease. Prednisone and vincristine were chosen because they have different modes of action, act rapidly, do not appreciably inhibit the regeneration of normal blood forming cells, and in combination, produce complete remissions in 90% of children with ALL. Neither are appropriate for prolonged maintenance of remission because of their serious cumulative side effects. Also, at diagnosis, ALL cells tend to have low DNA synthesis rates. Presumably, prednisone and vincristine are more appropriate at that time than drugs like methotrexate and mercaptopurine that act by interference with DNA synthesis.

The second phase is intensive chemotherapy after remission is achieved. The purpose is to reduce the remaining millions of ALL cells as quickly as possible to restrict the opportunities for them becoming resistant. The child's relatively normal health and blood cell formation after remission induction allows the administration of higher dosage and more drugs, especially those that depress blood cell formation and injure mucous membranes, than would have been tolerated initially. Also, by analogy with cell culture and from human experiments, it is reasonable to assume that the cell kill during remission induction stimulates DNA synthesis and replication of those remaining cells. This makes them more susceptible to the drugs we used for this phase: methotrexate, mercaptopurine and cyclophosphamide.

The purpose of the third phase is preventive or pre-emptive treatment of leptomeningeal leukaemia, including that portion which surrounds arteries and veins deep within the brain. As noted above both radiation therapy and the injection of methotrexate solution into the spinal fluid had been successful in the temporary relief of leptomeningeal leukaemia. Initially, we used radiotherapy because it provides uniform effects throughout the brain and spinal cord independent of spinal fluid circulation. Later, we combined radiation to the brain and multiple methotrexate injections into spinal fluid. (Note: After 1982, I used multiple injections of methotrexate plus two other anti-leukaemia drugs through all phases of treatment and avoided radiotherapy.)

The last phase of total therapy is continued chemotherapy with methotrexate, mercaptopurine and cyclophosphamide for two and a half to three years. The purpose is to eliminate residual "slow" ALL cells that might replicate only occasionally and might only be vulnerable to these drugs then. Previous experience had shown that stopping drug treatment within a short time after remission induction guaranteed prompt relapse.

The early studies of total therapy were fraught with many dangerous, difficult and often discouraging complications. Serious and often fatal infections by opportunistic microbes resulted from the severe suppression of immune response, often when autopsy demonstrated no evidence of leukaemia. Among the infections were *Pneumocystis carinii* pneumonia. We had the first reported epidemic in North America. Recurrent leptomeningeal relapse occurred despite preventive irradiation, causing debilitating neurological disease while the child remained otherwise free of leukaemia.

We also had a problem in human blood procurement for our children. All blood donation was commercial in Memphis. Beside the expense, many donors were at high risk for transmission of hepatitis. Fortunately, sailors and marines from a nearby base and local university students volunteered to be donors and came to our rescue.

Only the suffering of dying children, the family grief, the determination of the parents to find a cure, and the encouragement of the St Jude basic scientists kept us trying. The scientists berated us: "The ideas are correct; the problem is you expect an experiment to work right away." Parents pleaded: "We know our child will die but if you can learn something from our child that will help another child, please try."

One of the sustaining influences was the pioneering and successful basic research conducted by the young and enthusiastic staff. For examples, Allan Granoff and David Kingsbury opened new doors into molecular virology; Robert Webster demonstrated the origin of influenza epidemics in migratory birds, and George Cheung discovered an important calcium binding, protein-calmodulin. Luis Borella identified T-cell ALL, introducing the biological classification of ALL (see Chapter 3).

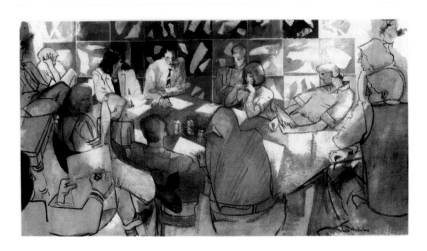

'*Weekly Co-Ordinating Meeting*' by Susan Macfarlane.

The staff of the Bone Marrow Transplant Unit hold regular meetings to plan and assess the treatment of all the patients in their care. "*The body language of each and every member helped to make this an interesting design.*" Oil on Canvas. 56 × 101.5 cm. (Courtesy of Euan and Angus Mackay and Dr Geoffrey Farrer-Brown).

Total Therapy Studies I to III

In the first three pilot studies, we learned that moderate dose leptomeningeal radiation was not effective in preventing leptomeningeal relapse. However, haematological remissions were longer than previously reported and seven of 37 children remained in complete remission for over three years. A difficult decision was made by the parents and ourselves to discontinue their chemotherapy. They were at risk of chronic toxicity and opportunistic infection while receiving it, and we had no other way to determine whether they were cured or in long chemotherapy dependent remission. More important, the children and their parents were ready to end the ordeal of treatment.

Approximately three to four months after chemotherapy was stopped, the children had numerous lymphoblasts in their bone marrows, suggestive of relapse. However, they felt better than they had in years and looked healthy so we observed them without restarting chemotherapy as the bone marrow gradually returned to normal appearance. We concluded that the high lymphoblast counts in the bone marrow represented an immune system rebound from the years of immune suppression by chemotherapy. Simultaneous rises in antibody responses to influenza vaccine that had been given during therapy supported this conclusion.

Four decades later, five of the seven survivors remain well and active. One died in 1979 of liver cancer caused by hepatitis B virus, most likely from a blood transfusion before this virus was identified and tested for. The other died from accidental drowning in 1978.

The long survival of one-fifth of children in studies I to III, continuously free of leukaemia and off therapy, indicated they were cured. ALL could no longer be considered incurable. Withholding treatment or palliative treatment alone was unacceptable. The challenge was to continue to increase the cure rate by developing more effective drugs and drug regimens, and finding better ways to prevent leptomeningeal relapse and to control infection.

Total Therapy Study IV

The high incidence of serious infections in studies I to III resulted in the deaths of patients in remission who were potentially curable. It also meant that chemotherapy was interrupted, allowing the resurgence of leukaemia cell replication and increased risk of relapse. In addition, the radiation to skull and spine depressed blood-forming cells so that tolerance of chemotherapy was lessened. Finally, a question was raised from mouse leukaemia studies whether the immune system might have a role in controlling leukaemia. Did full dosage chemotherapy in ALL depress a hypothetical host immune response to the ALL?

In Study IV, radiation therapy to the nervous system was withheld because it had not been effective in preventing leptomeningeal relapse. It was stopped in order to allow higher dosage of drugs. Full dosage of four drug continuation chemotherapy was compared with half dosage. The results demonstrated that full dosage was more toxic but remissions were longer, largely because of later and less frequent leptomeningeal relapse, which remained a major problem. We concluded that maximal dosage of drugs was more effective than lower dosage and contributed to the prevention of leptomeningeal relapse. It was obvious again that an effective way to prevent leptomeningeal relapse was essential to improving cure rates of childhood ALL. It was also apparent that better infection control to accommodate the immune suppression of maximal drug dosage was needed.

Total Therapy Study V

Another pilot study was begun in 1967 that encompassed two major changes. Radiation therapy dose was increased to what had been found adequate for the treatment of lymphoblastic brain tumours and it was confined to the cranium. To prevent leptomeningeal relapse in the spine and augment prevention in the brain, methotrexate was injected into the spinal fluid at three to four day intervals during radiation therapy. Secondly, two-week reinduction "pulses" of prednisone and vincristine were given periodically during continuation chemotherapy because of a report that it prolonged remissions in patients receiving mercaptopurine. Based on experience with studies I to III, the plan called for the stopping of treatment after three years of continuous complete remission.

At this time, I was fortunate to attract Dr Joseph Simone as Chief of Hematology. With Drs Rhomes Aur, Manuel Versoza, Luis Borella,

Charles Pratt, our radiotherapist Dr Omar Hustu, and members of the Nursing and Laboratory Staffs, Dr Simone soon organised and assumed leadership of the Total Therapy team.

Improved outcome was apparent within six months of initiating Study V. Of 35 consecutive children with ALL, 31 developed complete remission, only three of whom experienced leptomeningeal relapse, a five-fold reduction from previous studies. This was the first evidence that relapse at this site was preventable. Seven of the children had haematologic relapse. This was the lowest rate ever observed. Four decades later, one half of the children enrolled in study V remain alive and free of leukaemia (Fig. 8).

Study V confirmed the curability of childhood ALL and demonstrated the potential of cancer chemotherapy to cure cancer even when it has spread throughout the entire body. No cancer could be considered "hopeless" as long as drug development and strategic

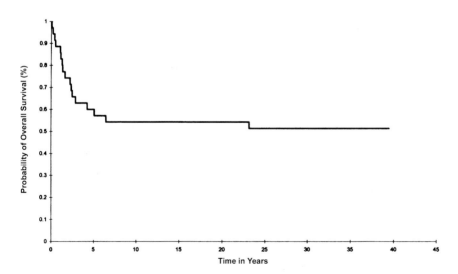

Fig. 8. Graph of survival of children with acute lymphoblastic leukaemia treated in Total Therapy V, 1967–1968. All children who survived for 8 years have survived for 40 years except for one who died from a radiation-related cancer. The plateau of survival indicates that the children were cured of leukaemia. Graph update was provided by Dr C-H Pui, St Jude Children's Research Hospital.

planning of its use alone or in conjunction with other treatment methods continued.

The results of this study were quickly accepted and the four-phase treatment plan implemented in many medical institutions and their cooperative groups after the presentation and publication of Study V results in 1971. In the USA, the national five year survival rate for childhood ALL rose from 5% for patients diagnosed in 1965 to 53% for 1975 patients.

Perhaps buoyed by the possibility of a cure for ALL and some other formerly fatal cancers, we moved on to total honesty with our children about prognosis, as suggested by Dr Myron Karon in his landmark publication, "Who's afraid of death on the leukaemia ward?" Later, we began to explain the treatment plan to the children as young as five years old and seek their written assent at the same time we sought consent from the parents.

Total Therapy Studies VI to VIII

Concern remained about using cranial radiation because of radiation encephalitis that occurred shortly after and its potential for eventually causing loss of brain function, brain tumours or other cancers in the radiation fields. We wondered if we could reduce the use of radiation.

In Study VI, from 1968 to 1970, a comparison was made between giving preventive radiation to the cranium and spine shortly after remission versus giving it only when closely monitored spinal fluid showed signs of early leukaemia. We might have compared a third option, periodic injection of methotrexate into spinal fluid but another institution reported that this had failed to prevent leptomeningeal relapse. I wish that we had included that comparison because our method of injecting drugs into spinal fluid was different and, I think, more effective.

An innovation in Study VI was the incorporation of daunomycin in the remission induction phase. This natural antibiotic isolated from a soil bacillus, combined with prednisone, had produced complete remissions in children with drug resistant ALL. Its most threatening toxicity is heart damage that accumulates and becomes permanent with high dose and prolonged use. Also, in an attempt to simplify treatment, which is one of our goals, the methotrexate, mercaptop-urine and cyclophosphamide during the continuation phase were taken orally instead of intravenously.

The results demonstrated that complete remission, survival and cure were significantly better and similar to those in study V for those who received the radiation before there was any evidence of leukaemia in the spinal fluid. The need for preventive leptomeningeal treatment was confirmed. No conclusion could be reached about the added benefit of daunomycin and it was usually omitted or min-imised in following studies because of its risk to the heart in growing children.

In Study VII, from 1970 to 1972, we compared two methods of preventive leptomeningeal treatment: cranial and spinal radio-therapy versus cranial radiotherapy and simultaneous injections of methotrexate into the spinal fluid. Both methods proved to be equally effective in most patients.

It was not until 1982 that the Pediatric Oncology Group led by Dr Pat Sullivan showed that preventive radiation was unnecessary for children whose spinal fluid was normal at diagnosis. Periodic injections into the spinal fluid of methotrexate combined with two other anti-leukaemia drugs throughout all phases of treatment were just as effective. Our experience over the past 35 years indicates that radiation therapy is a major factor in causing secondary cancer and impaired brain function in survivors of childhood ALL.

The question was raised about the problem of lowering dosage of individual drugs when they are combined. Was the advantage of combining drugs cancelled by the lower doses of the most effective and the consequent risk of inadequate tissue levels and pro-motion of drug resistance? Methotrexate was assumed to be the most effective, mercaptopurine the second most. To answer the question,

Study VIII was designed. Its continuation phase compared four different treatments: methotrexate alone; methotrexate and mercaptopurine; methotrexate, mercaptopurine and cyclophosphamide; and methotrexate, mercaptopurine, cyclophosphamide and a new drug, cytosine arabinoside. Cytosine arabinoside is a synthetic compound that inhibits the incorporation of an essential component into DNA. All of these drugs were given intravenously, except mercaptopurine, and all in the maximum tolerated dosage. As expected, doses had to be lower with increasing drug number in order to avoid lethal toxicity. A new drug was added to the remission induction in Study VIII, asparaginase. This enzyme, produced by bacteria, causes the depletion of the amino acid asparagine and the consequent reduction in protein synthesis.

The results showed that the methotrexate and mercaptopurine combination was superior to methotrexate in extending remission and survival. Addition of cyclophosphamide or cyclophosphamide plus cytosine arabinoside did not improve outcome. The superiority of a combination chemotherapy was confirmed but with the caveat that there might be a limitation of benefit when drugs of less effectiveness are added.

Studies VI to VIII were difficult because we were tempted to use all available anti-leukaemic agents in all patients. However, the risks of these agents, both the immediate and obvious and the later more subtle and uncertain, in growing children, were compelling reasons to conduct comparative studies to make certain the risks were proportionate to survival benefits. Not only the cure of leukaemia but normal growth and physical, emotional and mental health as adults were at issue. As more children were cured, the need for permanent follow up clinic visits and serial physical and psychological evaluation became more imperative.

Neuropsychological services were initiated in 1970 to meet the needs of the children and their families and to investigate neuropsychological effects of leukaemia and its treatment so that they could be factored into treatment choices. An interesting event occurred

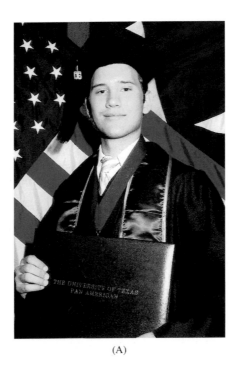

(A)

Fig. 9A.   Joseph, a survivor of ALL, treated at St. Jude. Joseph graduated from college summa cum laude. He is currently a medical student. Diagnosed with acute lymphoblastic leukaemia at age 3 years, his treatment plan avoided radiation therapy and simultaneous administration of methotrexate by vein and spinal fluid injection, the usual causes of brain impairment in children cured of leukaemia.

when federal support was requested for these studies. We were notified that a site visit by consultants was necessary. When the visitors arrived they had only one question: Do children survive ALL? After marvelling at the answer, the funds were recommended with enthusiasm.

During the early years at St Jude, my colleagues and I continued the search for a childhood ALL virus. Along the way, we developed a new method for quantitating mouse leukaemia viruses; searched for feline leukaemia virus in the patients; injected primates with ALL extracts, and determined the ultrastructure of human foetal thymus. But, like others, we were unable to identify a virus.

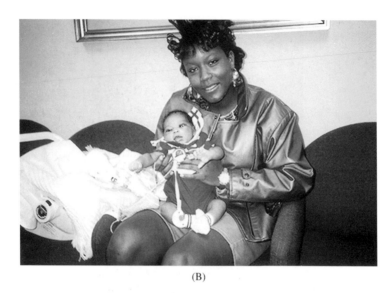

(B)

Fig. 9B.   Delysa, a survivor of T-cell ALL, treated at St. Jude and her son Anthony. When an adolescent, she had advanced T cell acute lymphoblastic leukaemia but became a mother four years after successful chemotherapy. Anthony is now a healthy 14 year old high school student and Delysa is an executive. Many people cured of leukaemia are parents. No evidence of leukaemia inheritance has appeared.

Curative Therapy of Childhood ALL, 1975–2008

During the past 35 years finding a cure for leukaemia has been the goal of treatment of childhood ALL. Four phase treatment plans similar to total therapy continue to be the usual standard of practice where circumstances permit. Teniposide, a natural compound extracted by Sandoz laboratories from the mandrake root, was found to have anti-leukaemia activity in childhood ALL and was introduced into some treatment plans in 1974. It interferes with DNA synthesis and cell replication by breaking DNA strands. One of its hazards, ironically, is increased risk of a secondary AML.

Since 1974, the advances in chemotherapy have been largely based on tailoring the treatment to different subtypes of ALL as identified by biological markers and extent of disease. T-cell ALL and Burkitt cell ALL are treated differently from the more common B cell precursor

ALL. Genetic characteristics are also used. For example, ALL with the abnormal #22 Philadelphia chromosome is characterised by a novel leukaemia-producing protein called BCR-ABL that results from the specific translocation of genes between chromosomes 9 and 22. For this reason, the patients are treated with a drug called imatinib mesylate (Gleevac), which targets that protein, in addition to the usual drug combinations for ALL. Synthesized by Swiss chemists and tested by Brian Drucker of Oregon, imatinib is the first effective anti-leukaemia drug specifically targeted to a leukaemia-producing protein.

I continued to participate in the study of childhood leukaemia and the care of children after departure from St Jude Children's Research Hospital in 1974. I initiated new research programs at other centers and continued to teach, treat patients and serve on national committees. Retired from paediatrics in 2001, I currently teach biological sciences at California Polytechnic State University in San Luis Obispo, California, and occasionally give lectures at the Children's Hospital of Los Angeles and elsewhere.

During the past 30 years, total therapy studies of ALL have been continued under the innovative and conscientious leadership of Dr Gaston Rivera and more recently Dr Chin-Hon Pui as St Jude Childrens' Research Hospital and opportunities for clinical investigation multiplied. My continued communication with them and their progress is a happy and enlightening experience (Fig. 10).

My last study of childhood ALL therapy was a pilot trial conducted from 1986 to 1994 at the University of Texas MD Cancer Center, Houston, and Driscoll Children's Hospital, Corpus Christi. It utilised genetic and immunological characteristics of ALL to determine the selection of treatment. Three-fourths of 150 consecutive unselected children were surviving eight years later. None received radiation therapy unless they experienced initial leptomeningeal relapse. In addition, the simultaneous injection of methotrexate into blood and into spinal fluid, which can be associated with brain damage, was avoided. As a consequence, none of the children experienced

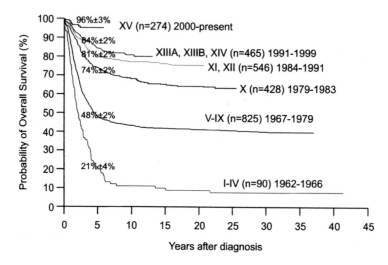

Fig. 10. Survival of children with ALL at St Jude 1962–2005. Graph of survival of children with acute lymphoblastic leukaemia treated at St Jude Children's Research Hospital on Total Therapy Studies I to XV from 1962 to 2005. Continued improvement in survival reflects the influence of experience, advances in supportive treatment and innovations in chemotherapy. Graph was provided by Dr C-H Pui and published in *New England Journal of Medicine*, 2006, 354: 166–178.

late neuropsychological sequelae due to leptomeningeal therapy, a nemesis in our earlier total therapy studies and in a concurrent national study. Few patients received daunomycin and even then, sparingly, in order to avoid another nemesis, heart disease.

Cure rates in the more affluent countries and communities have gradually improved during these past 35 years, but adjusting treatment to the different types of ALL and new drug combinations are only part of the reason. The remarkable increase of physicians and nurses trained to care for children with ALL and in facilities and resources for their diagnosis and treatment are major factors. Better infection control, such as prevention of *Pneumocystis pneumonia* by cotrimoxazole, and of varicella-zoster infection by immune globulin and immunization; new antibacterial and antiviral drugs; and more infectious disease specialists is another. The improvements in blood and platelet procurement and their screening for viruses are also a factor. Perhaps most important is the widespread acceptance that childhood ALL is curable and the consequent attitude that it must be cured.

Defining cure as 10-year survival five or more years after stopping chemotherapy, the current cure rate of childhood ALL at St Jude is approximately 80 percent (Fig. 10). The many multi-institutional cooperative groups studying the treatment of childhood ALL report cure rates of 70 to 75 percent. However, many children at high risk for treatment failure are excluded from group studies for various reasons, especially economic. Globally, cure rates vary from about 10 percent in impoverished communities and nations to about 70 percent in the prosperous countries. The reasons are well known and described. For most poor nations, communities and families, curative treatment of ALL is beyond reach despite international outreach programs conducted in numerous countries by St Jude and other children's cancer centres. The development of curative treatment of ALL is another advance that widens the gap between the available and the accessible in child health care.

Adults have been included in institutional and, in the USA, national collaborative treatment studies of ALL as well as AML along with children since the mid-1950s. The pioneer haematologist Max Wintrobe described the superior treatment response and survival of children in 1954. Although adult survival rates have improved considerably with curative treatment plans in the past three decades, they still remain less than those of children. One reason is the biological difference between childhood and adult ALL. For example, ALL with the traditionally less curable Philadelphia chromosome translocation subtype is five to six times more frequent in adults than children. Another reason is that children past infancy tend to be more resilient than adults and recover from disease and drug toxicity more readily. However, there is another factor. Recent comparison of adolescents and young adults with ALL with similar biological features demonstrate that their survival and cure are clearly superior when cared for in paediatric rather than adult leukaemia services. Is it Sidney Farber's teaching of "total care" long ago imbedded in most childhood cancer services that makes a difference?

"Spin-offs" of Total Therapy Studies

A "spin-off" is a valuable project or activity resulting from a research program that may have not been anticipated when the program began. The success in curing ALL and shedding of the hopeless label encouraged basic and clinical research to understand and find successful chemotherapy for many types of fatal cancer. This was especially true for adult cancer, which constitutes most of the total. In a way, this has distracted attention from the development of new drugs aimed specifically at childhood ALL, which is a very small market for drug manufacturers compared to adult cancers. Also, many cancer researchers began to see childhood ALL as an ideal model for their investigations so that the study of its biology and chemistry accelerated.

Early reports of curative treatment of ALL at St Jude helped stimulate institutional and national multi-institutional collaborative clinical studies of ALL and AML therapy in the United Kingdom, continental Europe, Japan, Australia and other nations. For example, the Medical Research Council studies in the UK and the Berlin-Frankfurt-Munster (BFM) studies in Germany have produced considerable information and new ideas regarding the biology of leukaemia. They have made remarkable advances in providing care of the children. French multi-institutional collaborative studies have shown how to cure the majority of children with the highly malignant Burkitt B cell leukaemia/lymphoma. Many of these treatment plans have been extended into Eastern Europe and often with modifications to less prosperous nations in Asia, Africa and South America. Some treatment plans have been imported into the USA and Canada by cooperative leukaemia study groups sponsored by the National Cancer Institute.

Another spin-off is the enkindled interest and research in the diagnosis, prevention and treatment of opportunistic infections by viruses, bacteria and fungi that do not ordinarily produce serious disease. The identification of the epidemic of *Pneumocystis pneumonia* among our children at St Jude led to research by Walter Hughes which demonstrated that this was a common inhabitant of the bronchi that became invasive in children whose immune response was depressed by malnutrition and anti-leukaemia drugs. The discovery by Dr Hughes in the 1970s that cotrimoxazole, in modest dosage, prevented *Pneumocystis pneumonia* reduced considerably its threat to children with cancer receiving chemotherapy. When the Acquired Immunodeficiency Disease (AIDS) epidemic was recognised in the 1980s, this was perhaps the first drug that extended the survival of patients with this disease by preventing this frequent cause of their death.

The serious and often fatal course of varicella-zoster virus infection (chicken pox and shingles) stimulated the development of varicella-zoster immune globulin (VZIG) to prevent or reduce the severity of these diseases, especially in persons with poor immune responses. The currently used varicella-zoster vaccine developed by Japanese researchers was tested and accepted in children with ALL many years before it was adopted for routine immunisation in all children.

When I began to see children with ALL at St Jude in the early 1960s, many had another disease: protein calorie undernutrition marked by growth failure and anaemia. Their tolerance of chemotherapy was seriously impaired. We initiated a paediatric nutrition program led by Paul Zee to address this problem in our patients. Later, a systematic community survey that he and his colleagues made in a low-income area of Memphis quantified widespread under-nutrition among newborn, infants and preschool children. With the participation of the community, we established a Child Nutrition and Health Program for pregnant and nursing mothers, infants and preschool children. This resulted in significant improvements in child growth and health in the community and became the model for the federal government's Women, Infants and Children (WIC) Program. Established in 1974, it now serves eight million mothers, babies and preschoolers in the USA and is called the government's most cost effective health programme.

An earlier spin-off of childhood leukaemia research is the use of "blood spots" for the diagnosis of genetic diseases such as phenylke-tonuria, a cause of mental retardation. In 1959, the late Dr Robert Guthrie and I were working together at Roswell Park Cancer Center to evaluate a new potential anti-leukaemia drug. He was using a bacterial assay method to determine the levels of the drug in the blood and urine of my patients, and so we spent many hours in conversation. At one point, we talked about mental retardation and its causes. I described phenylketonuria, which causes progressive mental retardation during the first year of life because of high levels of an amino acid that results from the genetic lack of an enzyme. After some thought, Dr Guthrie wondered if high levels of the amino acid could be identified in the newborn by his assay method. If so, the mental retardation might be prevented by omitting the amino acid from the baby's diet.

Thanks to my former mentor at Children's Hospital, Dr Mitchell Rubin, a place was found for him there and he was able to develop the first neonatal screening for this preventable disease. This was a landmark accomplishment. Mel Greaves and colleagues have been successful in using neonatal "Guthrie spots" for retrospective iden-tification of genetic markers signifying the pre-natal origins of ALL. Dr Guthrie ultimately made his contribution to ALL research long after his passing.

Current Challenges

Currently, several challenges in controlling childhood ALL are apparent. First by far is to identify precisely why children develop ALL in its various types and forms in order that it can be prevented. This is discussed in Mel Greaves' chapter.

Second is the need to resume the long neglected development of new and hopefully more specific, effective, easily administered drugs that are less toxic. Much of the cost of ALL therapy is related to drug administration and supportive care to overcome its toxicity. Simple, inexpensive curative treatment would allow logarithmic extension of its benefit to less affluent families, communities and countries. Drugs for childhood ALL cannot compete for attention in "free market" economies so that sizeable subsidies are needed. For example, the latest effective drug in childhood ALL, used in the 5 percent of children who have the Philadelphia chromosome type, was actually developed for adults with chronic myelocytic leukaemia, most of whom have this genetic anomaly.

Third is the need for more attention to eliminating chemotherapy that adds late hazards to the children with ALL without demonstrable and clinically significant advantages in restoring them to normal health, growth, development and life expectancy. Debilitation or death from cardiac failure, secondary leukaemia or other cancers, irreversible brain damage, permanently stunted growth, and organ failure are as tragic to the growing child or young adult as death from ALL. Close, careful follow up throughout the child's lifetime is essential to assessing these hazards and to quantifying human costs/benefits in order to guide treatment plans for newly diagnosed children.

Fourth is the need to limit the use of high cost, human and financial, treatments of ALL by methods that have failed to demonstrate higher cure rates than less costly treatment. An example is very high dose chemotherapy with or without total body irradiation followed by haematopoietic stem cell transplantation from a matched donor. Introduced in 1972 for children with relapsed ALL on the basis of anecdotal evidence, large comparative studies show that it is not more effective than chemotherapy in curing these children, only more toxic and expensive.

Finally is the need to extend curative treatment to all children by giving top priority to child health care for all families in all communities and nations. On one occasion, I made a professional visit to a state in Asia which had a very low per capita income. The children with ALL were receiving modern curative treatment and the cure rate was comparable to that of children in affluent states. Treatment was free and accessible to all children. When examined, I found that all measures of child health care in that state were generally comparable to those of affluent nations. The reason is that children are the first priority in that state, taking precedence over all other.

Attitude may be more important than affluence, not only in providing opportunity for cure to children with ALL, but in child health care delivery generally. This can be seen in the most wealthy nation, the USA, whose childrens' health ranks well below its wealth by international comparison, especially among low income families and in low income communities.

General References

1. CH Pui *Childhood Leukaemias*, 2nd edn. (Cambridge, Cambridge University Press) 2006.
   This book covers aspects of the diagnosis, treatment, biology and epidemiology of leukaemia, but is intended for a professional, medical/scientific audience.

Technical References

1. D Pinkel, Five year follow-up of "total therapy" of childhood lymphocytic leukaemia. *JAMA* **216**:648–652, 1971.
2. RJA Aur, Simone J, Hustu HO, Walters T, Borella L, Pratt C, and Pinkel D, Central nervous system therapy and combination chemotherapy of childhood lymphocytic leukaemia, *Blood* **37**:272–281, 1971.
3. R Manera, Ramirez I, Mullins J and Pinkel D, Pilot studies of species specific chemotherapy of childhood acute lymphoblastic leukaemia using genotype and immunophenotype, *Leukaemia* **14**:1354–1361, 2000.
4. C-H Pui and Evans WE, Treatment of acute lymphoblastic leukaemia, *N Engl J Med* **354**:166–178, 2006.

Editor's note. St. Jude is the patron saint for lost or hopeless causes. Donald Pinkel changed this designation at St. Jude Hospital, Memphis to 'hopeful causes' and all involved accepted it.

A SCIENTIST'S JOURNEY

Mel Greaves

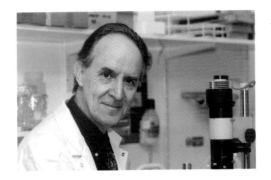

A SCIENTIST'S JOURNEY

Mel Greaves

I have been very fortunate to have spent most of my professional life doing research on childhood leukaemia, although as a young biologist, I could so easily have taken a different path. We all make these choices by accident or design and in my case, there were three compelling reasons. First, as a biology undergraduate at University College London (UCL), I was inspired by the Nobel Prize winner, Sir Peter Medawar. He made me believe that fascinating and challenging science could be coupled to important medical problems. Second, I discovered, pretty much by accident, around 1973, that childhood leukaemia was a problem crying out for some biological investigation. Clinicians, in particular, Donald Pinkel, were beginning to make real inroads into the therapeutic control of childhood leukaemia. However, it was evident that there was a wall of ignorance about the basis of leukaemias' clinical variability, its biology and causation. So, at that time, an opportunity existed and, serendipitously, immunology, the subject I had specialised in, provided a passport into that territory. Thirdly, and probably most significantly, at the time I was first confronted, in a London children's hospital, with pale and bald 2 to 5 year olds, in a leukaemia treatment ward, my own son and daughter were of the same age. Children at

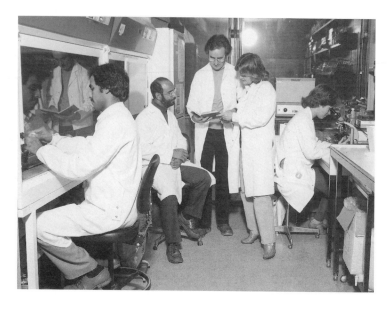

Fig. 11.   Lab shot 1980. Author in centre.

that age are very special indeed and it was impossible not to imagine, if only fleetingly, your own family in the same position. Hooked!

A year or so later, my decision was strongly endorsed by meeting a girl cured of leukaemia. She was at a special school for educationally subnormal children where my wife was working. Her father turned out to be a fellow biologist at UCL. More to the point, her leukaemia had been cured but her life had been effectively sabotaged physically and mentally, probably due to the irradiation to the brain, part of the treatment given. This brought home, vividly, the message that potentially curative therapy was an incredibly blunt instrument with harsh potential for collateral damage. And that much remained to be done.

Questions, Questions and Yet More Questions

"Progress in science consists not so much of finding the right answers... as of deciding what questions are sensible". Joseph Needham, 1936

Over the years, I have observed some superb scientists plying their trade. One thing they all seem to have had in common was the ability to synthesise the essence of a problem and come up with a laser-sharp but intrinsically simple question that goes straight to the heart of the matter. They ask the right question. And, invariably, the answer then appears to fall miraculously onto their plate. It may surprise lay readers to be told that this is not the way most scientists usually operate. This begs the question, of course, of what constitutes the right question. By definition, it has to address the central core of a problem and have the capacity, should it be answered, of resolving it. But in addition, it has to be a question that is ready or ripe for answering. As in music, sports, comedy and much else in life, timing is everything. A question that is ready for resolving is one where the essential framework of knowledge or understanding, though incomplete, is sufficiently mature that the experiment to test it can be intelligently designed. And, critically, there has to be the appropriate enabling technology. Creative ideas are the lifeblood of science but without technical innovation as the vehicle, nothing really moves ahead to convert speculation into fact. This has been especially true in the biology of leukaemia. So, in what follows as my personal narrative of a journey with leukaemia, the milestones are marked by questions as much as answers. These all relate ultimately to the same concerns that a parent of a patient would have: what exactly is leukaemia? What is wrong with the white blood cells? When did the white blood cells start to go wrong and what caused it? Or more pointedly: Why is it that my child has leukaemia?

It would be great if the answers to these important questions were to be simple:

— All leukaemias are one distinct disease entity with a single cellular defect — call it X.
— It is invariably caused by exposure to just one thing — call it Y.
— And it can be cured by a pill — call it Z.

You can make this kind of simplistic argument for many infectious diseases, tuberculosis for example. But leukaemia, and cancer in general, is just not like that. The challenge for any biologist tackling a biomedical problem of this kind is to take on board the inherent complexity, indeed to exploit it, but then to seek to distil out the major principles or consistent features involved.

You can only begin to do this if you are either naïve or very optimistic that such challenges are resolvable. You can only make progress if you are dogged, persistent and resilient to setbacks. In for the long haul, one step at a time. My apologies if this sounds like the attributes of a round-the-world lone yachtsman. It is not actually like that. Progress made in science does depend upon the imagination and drive of individuals. However, its execution and success is a highly social activity dependent upon teamwork, international collaborations and the constant reiterative search for consensual solutions. It demands the slow and careful construction of a plausible narrative. Leukaemia, AIDS, global warming … these are all similar types of challenge.

What follows is a personal narrative. It will appear self-referential and disguise the fact that everything that is done and every advance that is made exploits, to some extent, knowledge and insight provided by other fellow travellers.

Who's Who?

As outlined in the introductory chapter, for a hundred years acute leukaemias have been divided into two distinct types defined by simple, anatomical features of the cells visible down a microscope of modest magnification. Lymphoid-looking or myeloid-looking large (blast) cells gives us acute lymphoblastic leukaemia (ALL) and acute myeloblastic leukaemia (AML). These correspond to the two major types of white cells in our blood. For a long time, these two types of leukaemias were each treated clinically as if they were homogeneous disease entities. For someone, coming from the research field

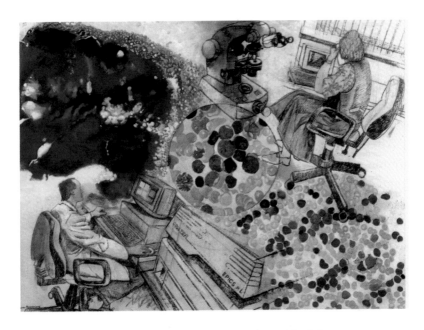

'*Typing the Leukaemic Cells*' by Susan Macfarlane.

"*I am shown amazing colours and shapes under the microscope and must try to do them some justice.*" To confirm that a child has leukaemia a bone marrow examination is essential. A Consultant Haematologist studies small samples of bone marrow smeared onto glass slides and then stained to assess the degree of marrow infiltration by leukaemic cells. The appearance down the microscope of a bone marrow infiltrated by acute lymphoblastic leukaemia, with the leukaemic cells stained blue, is shown in the painting at three different magnifications; low power top left, middle power bottom right and high power in the centre. One of the cells at 8 o'clock in the latter group is dividing, known as mitosis. The other member of the laboratory staff in the painting uses a flow cytometer which sorts the leukaemic cells according to any surface 'markers' present. The leukaemic cells have previously been reacted with a large series of fluorescent 'marker' proteins, or antibodies, which bind to any specific 'markers' present on the surface of the leukaemic cells. It is the identification of the specific 'markers' on the leukaemic cells which allows the leukaemia to be accurately typed. Oil on Canvas. 100×135 cm. (Courtesy of Euan and Angus Mackay and Dr Geoffrey Farrer-Brown).

of lymphocyte biology, such as myself, it was, a 'no-brainer' to ask exactly what kind of cells they were and how they might relate to the normal developmental biology and cellular hierarchy of the blood cell system. In the early 1970s, we already had the immunological tools to ask that question, as did just one or two other teams, in Paris and at

St. Jude in Memphis. It quickly became apparent that ALL, the major type of leukaemia in children, could be subdivided into two major lineages — T- and B-cell leukaemia which corresponded to immature cells or precursors in those two normal lymphocyte lineages. We were able to classify ALL then into T precursor (T) ALL and the more common (~75%) variant, B precursor or common (c) ALL (see Fig. 3 in introductory chapter). We were also able to generate, for the first time, antibodies that specifically identified cALL. A third infrequent (5%) subtype of ALL was prevalent in infants and of indefinite lineage but was later found to be a very primitive B lineage progenitor (pro-B ALL). A final fourth subtype was very rare (~2%) and had a mature B-cell phenotype.

The consequences of these relatively straightforward descriptive observations were considerable. Firstly, they led to the establishment of a national immuno-diagnostic service for childhood ALL in the United Kingdom. This referral centre used panels of discriminatory antibodies coupled with what was at the time a very novel automated single cell flow system using laser light to identify cells. These methods are used throughout the world today for the diagnosis and classification of leukaemia. Secondly, we were able to exploit the ongoing clinical trials for leukaemia in the 1970s to demonstrate that these subtypes had different prognostic outcomes. cALL was found to have a relatively good outcome, while pro-B infant ALL and B ALL had very poor outcomes. The treatment was subsequently modified or tailored to the various subtypes. Thirdly, these first tentative steps into the biology of childhood ALL suggested that very immature blood cells somehow become arrested in their normal development. Years later, we learned more about the biochemical mechanism that traps cells in this state of continuous proliferation. To me, at that time, this was redolent of the Queen's comment to Alice:

> *'Now, here, you see, it takes all the running you can do, to keep in the same place'*
> (The Red Queen to Alice in *Through the Looking Glass* by Lewis Carroll)

After classifying more than 1500 cases of childhood ALL in the UK, we found out the peak age of incidence for cALL was two to five years old. This peak (see Fig. 4 in introductory chapter) of leukaemia incidence in children became something of a personal obsession. Surely the peak was pertinent to the natural history of ALL in children and especially to its etiology? To explore this further, we undertook a rather ambitious plan in the early 1980s to similarly subclassify childhood ALL in many different centres throughout the world to see how universal these age matched subtypes were.

An international consortium was set up with colleagues in the Far East, Brazil, Chile, South Africa and other countries. Essentially, the results obtained in other countries was similar to that in the UK. However, the incidence of cALL in South African black children and Mapuche Indians of Chile was around 10-fold less. They had no marked 2–5 year peak age of incidence. This was a tantalising finding and was a fit with something else. This peak of incidence of childhood ALL was most apparent in the developed or affluent countries. Epidemiological registry data suggested that this peak of incidence of ALL emerged in the UK and USA between 1920 and 1940. However, it appeared later in Japan (1960s) and later still in

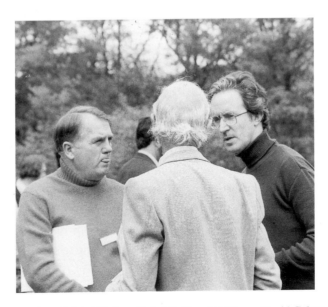

Fig. 12.   The author (right) with Don Pinkel (left) and Professor David Galton (centre) at a conference in Wilsede, Germany (1982).

China and in US black children (1970s). There were potentially trivial explanations for this: the disease might be underdiagnosed in certain social or geographic settings, and/or children might have died of pre-emptive infection before their leukaemia was recognised. However, the incidence of ALL but not AML appeared to be associated with affluence. With this in mind, I came up with a speculative idea of what the predominant cause of the major subtype of childhood ALL might be — and then spent much of the next 20 years trying to validate it. More on that later. But first, back to the beginning.

When Does it Start: Early Beginnings?

For common adult cancers, there are epidemiological clues to suggest that the malignant clone usually evolves over many years or decades, mostly in a clinically covert state in unsuspecting patients. Childhood cancers such as acute leukaemia clearly cannot take that long for the problem to surface. For a minority of cancers in children, bilateral tumours of the eye being the best example, their diagnosis early in life reflects the fact that they are kick-started by the inheritance of a mutant gene. This is very rare in leukaemia. So, for a child aged between two and five years old suffering from leukaemia, when is the cancer initiated? The production of white blood cells begins very early during the development of the unborn child — around six to seven weeks in the embryo. The white blood cells are formed first around the major aortic blood vessel, then, in the liver of the developing foetus. Eventually, blood production shifts to the bone marrow, continuing in this tissue after birth and indeed throughout life. So, in theory, leukaemia could begin anytime from the sixth week of gestation in pregnancy. A more tractable idea might be that it could start sometime before birth. I certainly was not the only one to consider this possibility. The problem, as always, was how to ask the question. Some twenty or more years ago, the Director of the Leukaemia Research Fund charity, Gordon Piller, said to me "Well, why don't you just screen hundreds of newborn babies for leukaemic cells?"

Quite so, but at the time, it just wasn't technically feasible. But the question wouldn't go away and a solution was eventually found.

Twins Show the Way

A key step was the acquisition of a sensitive and specific test for numerically rare leukaemia cells. The chromosomal, molecular abnormalities in leukaemia cells provide just the right marker for such a test. Research in many different laboratories, beginning in the 1980s and still continuing today, has identified a plethora of chromosomal alterations and subtle DNA changes or mutations in leukaemia cells — more than 200 in all. The particular constellation of genetic errors in any patients' leukaemic cells has a major impact on the response to therapy. Indeed, they are probably the main determinant of the eventual outcome since they exert a profound influence on drug sensitivity. For this reason, genetic profiling is now becoming the diagnostic method of choice for sub-classification of leukaemia. Additionally, there is much excitement and capital investment in the idea that the mutant genes of cancer cells might be the Achilles heel providing ideal specific targets for therapy. This idea has led to some success in the treatment of chronic myeloid leukaemia in adults.

Fortunately, a few of these manifold genetic changes are predominant or common. The leukaemic cells from many children with the same subtype of leukaemia, say cALL, will have what appears to be the same chromosome change and underlying molecular lesion or mutation (and therefore similar clinical response). But at the very precise level of DNA sequence changes, each mutation of the leukaemic cells is completely unique. This enabled us to design molecular probes that would only bind to and thus identify the abnormal genes of leukaemic cells of individual patients, even when these are incredibly few in number. We should then be in business for very sensitive detection of leukaemic cells. But were we? How can we *back*track in time with a patient that is already diagnosed with leukaemia? Just weeks before being diagnosed with ALL the patient will have appeared to have been a healthy and perfectly normal child. How can you find out what happened five years before?

The answer came from an unexpected source. In the early 1980s, I was running the national diagnostic service for the biological classification of childhood leukaemia linked to the ongoing MRC clinical trials. Over a period of two weeks, we had two bone marrow samples arrive for screening from the same hospital Great Ormond Street Hospital in London (GOSH) and with the same surname. I thought this might be a repeat sample on the same patient so I telephoned a clinical colleague only to be told that, no, they were from identical twins, both of whom had ALL. I had never heard of such a double diagnosis before and was intrigued enough to look into past clinical reports of twins with leukaemia. I discovered that the first such twin pair was recorded in Germany in 1880. Since that time, there had been around 50 or so such cases reported, all of the same sex and likely to have been identical twins. During the 1960s and 1970s, there was a flurry of debate on this topic and various possible explanations profered. The most likely explanation was that the twins, being genetically identical (they are derived from the splitting of a single fertilised egg), had coinherited the same leukaemia predisposition gene. But this seemed at odds with the fact that a high rate of disease concordance was not seen for other paediatric cancers and there was little or no evidence for a greatly increased risk of leukaemia in non-identical twins (who are derived from two fertilised eggs) or in siblings (who still share 50% of their genes) or families generally. One alternative and radical suggestion appealed as very plausible. This was based on the recognised fact that most (though not all) identical twins, whilst in the womb, share a single placenta with vascular connections between them. The consequence of this is that the twins literally share each other's blood and are blood cell chimaeras. It is this arrangement, something of an accident of nature, that gives rise to some of the serious medical complications of twinning. It was speculated that both the twins will have leukaemia due to spread from one twin to the other, via their shared blood supply. But how can you show that two twins share the *same* clone of leukaemia cells derived from just one of them? There was no satisfactory way of answering this question in the 1980s. However, if we had our hands on the precise chromosomal change that actually initiated the disease, then this might be resolvable. We began a very slow process of collecting samples on twin pairs from a network of colleagues from all over the world. This kind of project takes time. If the chance of any child having leukaemia is around one in two thousand, then the probability of having a pair of twins in a family, both with leukaemia, is something like one in two million.

I should interject something personal here. Lest I sound like a cold blooded scientist, let me recall how I felt about pairs of twins with leukaemia. In a nutshell, schizophrenic. On the one hand, I was excited that we might have a crucial lead in discovering how leukaemia develops. On the other hand, I felt very sad for the parents of children with leukaemia and even more so for parents of twins with leukaemia: a double burden. As we progressed in our research, we uncovered the world's only triplet pairs with leukaemia. How bad can things get? In one set of triplets from Manchester, the two identical twins who shared a single placenta both had ALL, the non-identical twin with her own placenta was healthy. In the other set of triplets from the Slovac Republic, all three girls shared the same placenta and, tragically, all three developed ALL.

We first studied three very informative twin pairs of infants with the pro-B variant of ALL These came from Chile (see Fig. 13(A)), Guatemala (via St Jude Children's Hospital, Memphis) and Scotland. By that time, we already knew that a particular DNA change or gene alteration was common in infant ALL. The gene involved had the code name *MLL* and we had already shown that in a set of unrelated infant patients with this leukaemia that the precise position in the DNA sequence of the gene where it was damaged was unique to each patient. Therefore, specific probes could be developed.

The excitement for me here came not so much from the answer, which I sensed was obvious, but from the realisation that the question that we always wanted to ask could be addressed. Seeing for the first time that the leukaemic cells from each pair of twins shared exactly the same unique mutation was one of those rare eureka moments. The critical point here was that such a unique mutation was not coin-herited by the twins, and could only have happened once only in a single cell. The only credible explanation was that in these pairs of twins, leukaemia was initiated by a gene mutation in one cell in one foetus with the resultant proliferating clone of cells spreading, via their shared blood, to the co-twin in the womb. Over the next ten years, we confirmed this shared single cell or clonal, pre-natal origin of childhood leukaemia in many other twin pairs with different chromosomal, DNA-based lesions; they all shared the same single initiating event or mishap in their blood cell DNA.

These twin experiments were not without clinical consequence. The type of leukaemia prevalent in infants is highly malignant and the prognosis is very poor. What happened in two of our pairs of twins (including the pair featured Fig. 13A) was this: one twin of each pair was unwell and clinically diagnosed with leukaemia. They were treated accordingly but unfortunately, they did not survive. At the same time, the co-twin was clinically well and the blood picture was normal. However, we decided to look at the bone marrow of the healthy co-twin. What we saw there were unmistakable signs of leukaemia. The co-twin had the same leukaemia, in molecular signature, as the sibling but at a less advanced stage. These children were then given chemotherapy and are alive and well today. We presume that it is because we were able to detect the disease and start chemotherapy early enough.

Now, leukaemia in twins is no different biologically or clinically from leukaemia in non-twinned children. There just happens to be two developing babies nourished by the same placenta. It seemed reasonable to assume that if leukaemia starts before birth in the twin context, the same must hold for other non-twinned children with leukaemia.

But there was a catch, a serious caveat to consider. For twin children in the peak of incidence of ALL at two to five years of age, the concordance rate is not 100% but 10%. This translates to a risk of around 1 in 10 for a twin whose identical twin sibling already has leukaemia. This is still a 100-fold increase in risk compared to another, non-twinned sibling. It could be argued therefore that concordant pairs of twins are very special and that for the 90% that are *dis*cordant for leukaemia, i.e. only one of the pair has leukaemia, and similarly for the majority of non-twinned children, leukaemia was *not* initiated before birth.

Fortunately, a solution to this conundrum emerged.

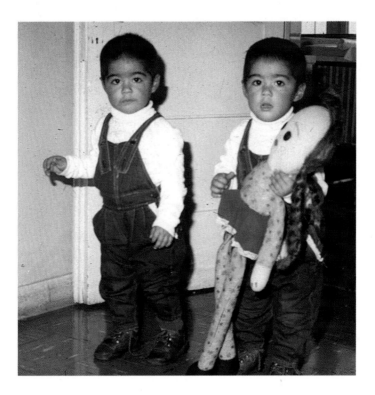

Fig. 13A. Twin patients. Both these infants, from Chile, had acute leukaemia and were the first twin pair in which we demonstrated a common pre-natal origin of the disease, in 1993. (with permission of parents)

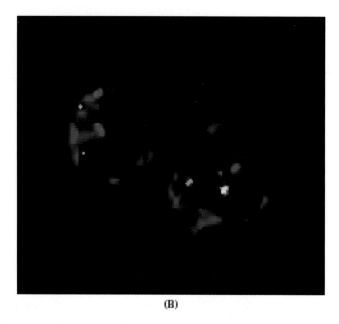

(B)

Fig. 13B. Visualising abnormal genes by I-FISH. I-FISH: *F*luorescence *I*n *S*itu *H*ybridisation to identify specific genes combined with (I) immune antibodies (blue) to recognise cell type. Two cells from a normal baby's cord blood. Cell on the left is normal immature B cell: 2 red genes, 2 green genes. Cell on the right has red/green fusion (=yellow), the marker of chromosome exchange of DNA (=translocation) and leukaemia initiation.

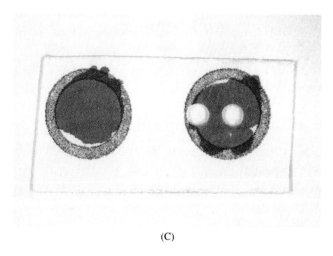

(C)

Fig. 13C. Neonatal blood spots (Guthrie cards). Cards with single blood drops taken in the first week of life: a vital, archived source of blood cell DNA. This image is two times real size.

Forensic Blood Spots

Readers will know that from a single spot of blood found at the scene of a crime or on the clothes of a suspect, forensic scientists can identify the source of that blood using very sensitive DNA 'fingerprinting' methods. It turns out that we were able to do something very similar to this for leukaemia. Over a beer at a conference in Germany sometime around 1995, I was telling colleagues that what I desperately needed was an accessible source of blood from newborns. One obvious source was the cord or even placenta itself that was usually discarded (my daughter's placenta was used to fertilise the garden roses). But, ideally, what was needed was a source of routinely stored blood, including that from individuals who eventually develop leukaemia. A clinical colleague pointed out the existence of so-called Guthrie cards (see Fig. 13(C)). These are literally cards onto which a single drop of blood is collected, usually by a district nurse, by heel prick from the baby's foot in the first week of life. The dried neonatal blood spot is archived, often for many years, and is routinely used to screen for an inborn metabolic defect called PKU. This was just what we needed! Don Pinkel told me that when Dr Guthrie was developing the idea of the blood spot cards 50 years ago, his paediatric department chief told him that he should stop his research as it had no possible relevance to leukaemia. A nice twist in the story as it has transpired.

In the 1980s, it was discovered that the DNA from the white blood cells in the dried blood spot remains relatively intact. It was thus possible to extract the DNA and test it for inherited mutations involved in, for example, sickle cell anaemia or cystic fibrosis. In such situations, every white cell in the spot (some 30,000 in all) will have carried the mutation making detection relatively easy. This was especially so when the polymerase chain reaction (PCR) method was invented by the Nobel Prize-winning and the somewhat maverick scientist, Kary Mullis. This technique can generate millions of copies of pieces of DNA or genes present at extremely low levels.

But the argument we had to make was more demanding. It went like this:

IF	we are right about the origins of leukaemia transmission from twin to twin *in utero*, then leukaemic cells had to be present in their blood at some time (and not just in their liver or bone marrow where they are probably spawned);
and IF	leukaemia in twins is biologically exactly the same as leukaemia in most non-twinned children;
THEN	the leukaemic mutation might be detectable in the archived blood spot of a patient with leukaemia;
PROVIDED	that the mutation used as a marker for the leukaemic cells really was the first or initiating genetic change, rather than a later (post-natal) alteration;
and IF	the number of leukaemia cells in the blood at birth, and several years before the disease was diagnosed, was, at the very least, present at more than 1 cell per single blood drop — or 1 in 30,000 white cells;
and IF	the PCR test is working optimally to detect very few mutant cells (not a given).

This looks like a rather too long list of ifs and buts. But this is how science operates. The art form is using some judgement to decide if what's being proposed as a question is too much of a long shot or is worth a serious punt. It was, in this case, the latter. It turned out that in most cases of leukaemia in children aged anything between a few months old and 12 years, we could indeed identify the unique leukaemia mutation in their blood spots, thereby proving unambiguously that leukaemia usually starts before birth. Whether it always does so is another matter. It may not, we cannot tell. And, just to make it very clear: the leukaemia mutations in the blood spots, as in the twin cells, are early acquisitions in the developing baby's blood cells. They are not inherited from parents.

Cords Galore

The very satisfying blood spot result carried another important implication. This was that in the context of the nine out of ten twin pairs that were *dis*cordant for leukaemia, it was likely that the twin who remained healthy harboured leukaemic cells generated and shared before birth, but that some trigger and associated secondary, but still essential, DNA mutations were absent. This accorded with a two-hit model that I had conjured up as a speculative scenario for leukaemia development many years before. This postulated that a minimum of two independent DNA or gene mishaps/mutations in a blood cell, one before birth, one after, had to occur for acute leukaemia to emerge clinically. We have, in fact, only recently been able to show that leukaemic cells with just the one or first genetic "hit" are indeed present and persistent in the blood of a healthy child whose co-twin has ALL (see Epilogue at end of chapter). The two-hit model was important to endorse not least because it would identify two distinct time windows, one before and one after birth when critical events and, possibly, critical exposures might be causing leukaemia. But then the twins' observations prompted an additional thought. If in nine times out of ten, hit number two didn't happen to the second twin already primed for leukaemia by hit one, how often does leukaemia arise before birth but never mature to a diagnosis? Compared to, that is, with the risk of 1 in 2000 for the disease itself. Leukaemia is a rare disease but is its initiation in the womb rare? This is not an esoteric or academic point. Epidemiologists trying to get at the cause of a disease such as childhood leukaemia regard it as a relatively rare occurrence.

In order to answer the question, we then did at long last what Gordon Piller had, with some prescience, suggested we do about 20 years previously. We screened several hundred cord bloods taken at birth of normal healthy babies for the presence of leukaemic cells carrying specific leukaemia-causing chromosome changes — the same genetic changes shared by twins and present in neonatal blood spots of patients with leukaemia. This experiment was a real headache logistically, ethically and technically. So, that was another slog, this

M. Greaves

time for around four years in all. But eventually, we got there in 2002. We could, for the first time, visualise the covert mutation harbouring leukaemic cells (Fig. 13(B)). And the striking numerical result was this: for every single child with leukaemia there appears to be around 100 children born with a leukaemic clone of cells on board but which never sees the light of day, clinically speaking. This finding should change the way we think about leukaemia; at least it did for me. As many as 1 in 20 children may lead perfectly normal, healthy lives, unaware of the presence since birth of what we now call the *pre*-leukaemic population. Cells latent with malignant potential but lacking the full credentials. Just one percent of children harbouring such clones go on to develop ALL.

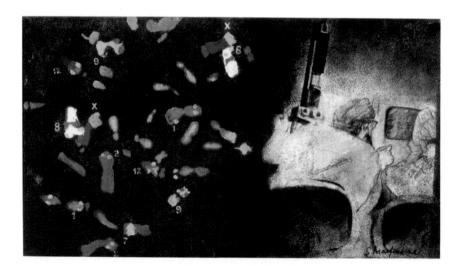

'Cytogenetics: A Lesson on Typing the Chromosomes' by Susan Macfarlane.
"*A Consultant Scientist is showing a trainee the work done in the Cytogenetics laboratory.*"
Depicted are the microscope, computer and a small square representation of a photo of chromosomes printed against a black background that shows up the luminous colours of the fluorescent DNA probes which identify specific gene defects. Study of chromosome pattern is very helpful in identifying different types of leukaemic cells and predicting the likely response to treatment. Oil on Canvas. 24 × 45.5 cm. (Courtesy of Euan and Angus Mackay and Dr Geoffrey Farrer-Brown).

Making Babies and Playing Roulette?

Whatever causes the first hit in the womb has to be common; indeed, there is a technical argument, not detailed here, that says the causative exposure has to be ubiquitous or present in all of us as developing babies. My own view reflects a decided preference (or bias perhaps) that I have towards the evolutionary explanations for our vulnerability to medical mishaps. Contrary to what some like to believe, we have not been intelligently engineered by millions of years of evolution to near perfection. The slow evolutionary process, driven predominantly by natural selection of random genetic variations, cobbles the best available solutions together. The inevitable consequence is that we have manifold imperfections, compromises and trade-offs on board. It's nothing short of amazing to me that a normal baby develops from a fertilised egg. But the error rate is high; many early embryos die spontaneously, around 1 percent of us are born with abnormalities and all of us are carrying mutations of one sort or another. This really shouldn't be surprising given the magnitude of the task of making something as complex as a human baby. The architectural challenge of assembling a fully functional baby's body involves massive cell migration and cell death, three-dimensional tissue assembly and billions of rounds of proliferation that require faithful copying, in each cell, of the entire genetic code in the face of constant assault by DNA-damaging products of our internal, metabolic processes. My view is that many childhood leukaemias, and probably most paediatric cancers, may be initiated as a consequence of this natural, error-prone process. That's not to say that the process is not susceptible to outside influence. The fact that babies born with greater than anticipated average weight have significantly increased risk of leukaemia may indicate that maternal diet can influence the number of cells at risk from those otherwise spontaneous events in the developing baby. It may seem counter-intuitive that such a critical process as making a healthy baby should frequently generate mutant premalignant clones. Surely, you might say, evolution itself should have weeded out this sloppy control? It probably would have done so if "one hit" had been enough to produce a lethal cancer. But that's the point: one hit is necessary to get the pathological process moving but it is insufficient and in itself harmless. Clearly what really matters, the real bottleneck, is whatever triggers the conversion of the silent pre-leukaemic clone to full blown leukaemia, usually at around two to five years of age at the peak. So what might that be?

What's the Trigger?

The quest for an understanding of the cause of childhood leukaemia is a very long-running saga — 100 years or more. To be frank, we still do not have a definite answer. The explanations paraded are legion. Here is a selection of postulated causal exposures from the published epidemiological literature (Table 1).

Beggar's belief, doesn't it? There are several problems here. One is, with the best will in the world, epidemiologists haven't been able to define the question well enough and have found it difficult to design large, statistically robust and well controlled studies. For a

Table 1.   Postulated causal exposures.

- Car exhaust fumes
- Pesticides
- Ionising radiation
- Non-ionising electromagnetic fields
- Electric fields
- Vitamin K injection at birth
- Hot dogs or hamburgers (depending on whether the patient was in California or Colorado)
- Domestic animals
- Organic dust from cotton, wool or synthetic fibres
- Natural light deprivation through melatonin disruption
- Artificial, fluorescent light exposure in hospital neonatal care units
- Parental cigarette smoking
- Maternal medicinal drug taking (during pregnancy)
- Maternal alcohol consumption (during pregnancy)
- Chemical contamination in drinking water
- Infections

long time, they assumed that childhood leukaemia was one disease with one cause awaiting to be discovered. This has zero chance of being correct. It is not like lung cancer and cigarette smoking; and even lung cancer cause is not quite as simple as it seems.

What the biology suggests is this: that there are several very different kinds of leukaemia and the related cancer, lymphoma. We know that leukaemia can sometimes be caused by high dose irradiation (the Hiroshima bomb experience), by some chemicals (benzene), and by particular viruses (one called EBV for a type of childhood lymphoma, another called HTLV-1 in adult lymphoma/leukaemia in West Africa and Japan). In domesticated animals (cats, cattle and chickens), common leukaemias and lymphomas are mostly caused by specific viruses. Acute leukaemias in children and adults can also arise, most ironically, as a consequence of the DNA-damaging properties of cancer treatment drugs: so cured of one cancer but leukaemia arriving as "collateral damage". In these examples, leukaemias are usually of particular subtypes and are clearly linked to specific and unusual insults or exposures.

So the lesson from this is that there is no universal or single cause of childhood leukaemia. But maybe major and minor or rare causes allied to different types of blood cell cancers. The other message from biology is that leukaemia, as I've tried to describe, develops in discrete stages. This immediately posits the distinction between what might cause initiation (in the womb) and what triggers the disease later in life, more proximate to a diagnosis. I've already explained why I believe that the trigger after birth is the key practical question. But what might that trigger be?

In 1988, I published a highly speculative article outlining what I thought might be a major causal mechanism for childhood ALL. The motivation was finding an explanation for the striking peak incidence of common (B-cell precursor) ALL at two to five years of age that appeared to track with affluence in society. It went like this:

— Childhood ALL develops in two discrete stages or mutational hits, one before, one after birth. The first "hit" results in a persistent but clinically silent premalignant clone of leukaemic cells.
— The prenatal events, chromosome changes, were effectively accidental or spontaneous, i.e. no external causes.
— The post-natal "trigger" was predominantly an abnormal immunological response to one or more common infection(s) that could be viral, bacterial or either. The striking peak incidence of ALL between two and five years of age is then a reflection of the timing of the trigger itself, which effectively precipitates the disease.

As I've outlined above, our subsequent research showed that the minimal two-hit model was essentially correct. But what about an infectious trigger?

The idea that childhood leukaemia might be caused by infection itself was certainly not new. Back in the early part of the 20th century, clinicians considered this a possibility and observed that the incidence peak at two to five years of age coincided with the timing of common infections such as measles. They were, however, put off the track of an infectious origin by the lack of evidence and, in part, because it was apparent that leukaemia didn't transmit from person to person. Some, however, were probably on the right track, or rather the track I believe is leading to an answer:

> *"We incline on our evidence to the belief that the solution of the problem of leukaemia lies rather in some peculiar reaction to infection than in the existence of some specific infective agent".*
> (J Poynton, H Thursfield and D Paterson, Great Ormond Street Hospital for Sick Children, London, **1922**)

Parenthetically, when I was cogitating these ideas in the mid 1980s, I had an informal meeting with the then Secretary of State for Health, the very youthful Dr David Owen who was himself trained as a doctor. His son had been diagnosed with ALL and he told me he had a strong suspicion that it was triggered by a measles attack. Very interesting, I thought. There has, on the other hand, never been any credible evidence to support a *direct* role of infection, i.e. a virus that infects blood cells and converts them into leukaemic derivatives. As scientists discovered in the 1970s that leukaemias in cattle, cats and chickens was caused by particular viruses, the instinctive reaction was: if it's true for domesticated animals, then why not domesticated humans? With colleagues in Glasgow, we've spent ten years using every available molecular probing test to identify an offending, specific virus in childhood leukaemia cells. It does not appear to exist and almost certainly does not exist.

When, in 1988, we suggested an infectious trigger might be the cause of leukaemia, an insightful epidemiologist, Leo Kinlen, came up independently with a similar explanation. In his case, he was concerned to explain the cluster of cases of childhood leukaemia around the nuclear reprocessing plant at Sellafield, in the area of Cumbria, UK. Folklore and conventional wisdom insisted that this cluster must be caused either by exposure of young children to radiation leaks (which certainly occurred) or that children were inheriting leukaemia-predisposing mutations from their dads who worked at the reprocessing plant and themselves had been exposed to radiation. Kinlen suggested a radically different alternative. The village of Seascale next to the Sellafield plant was an unusual social artefact and rapid mixing of families brought together from all over the UK for occupational reasons may have resulted in the contagious spread of a leukaemia-causing virus. Over the following 15 years or so, Kinlen and colleagues investigated more than a dozen other situations of "sudden population mixing", including the construction of rural new towns and army camps. In each situation, they documented a transient increase in childhood leukaemia shortly after the "mixing" occurred. Kinlen favours a specific virus, as found in animal leukaemias, but this, as I've indicated, is unlikely to be the case.

Marked clusters of childhood leukaemia are not common but they have been described several times. One of the first was in the district of Niles, a suburb of Chicago in 1957 to 1960 and the latest is the most marked of all: 14 cases over four years where only one would normally be anticipated. And where is this? Around a "top gun" naval air base in the small town of Fallon, Nevada. The answer is obvious particularly if you've seen the Hollywood movies "*A Civil Action*" and "*Erin Brockovich*"? Surely it must be the leaking, carcinogenic jet fuel? Scientists are trying to study the cluster but the place is crowded out with litigation lawyers and filmmakers. The best bet for Fallon is that it is some unusual immune response to infection related to population mixing. But proving the real cause of a cluster such as this is extremely difficult.

Paradox, or Grandma's Wisdom?

If infection is in some way responsible for triggering ALL, then why on earth should it be linked to affluence; surely the opposite should apply — more proverty equals more infection?

It comes back to the unanticipated consequences of evolution to which we are inevitably subjected. The immune system of humans is extraordinarily dynamic. Rather like the brain, it is not born hard-wired but learns, and its component parts become architecturally net-worked, by experience in early life; in the case of the immune system by natural infection. Paradoxically, it actually needs infection to set it up for proper function and if deprived of these "priming" expo-sures, it malfunctions. The cellular basis of this exposure-dependent design is relatively well defined in mice, less so in humans. The corollary is this: the way the system has evolved or adapted is to *anticipate* infection very early in life, in the womb and shortly after birth. Moreover, evolution has continually refined the system by Darwinian natural selection. Survivors of past infectious plagues were almost certainly the accidental genetic beneficiaries of more potent anti-infectious responses. So imagine now a Victorian slum-dwelling infant is transported by a tardis to the 21st century Western society city suburb. Where are the necessary infections? Largely erad-icated of course. And with some considerable benefit since infant and childhood mortality from infectious causes has declined dramatically. But maybe at a cost. A poorly primed immune system can react inappropriately later, say when children mix with their peers at school and inevitably share common infections. Triggering leukaemia via an unregulated immune response in susceptible individuals could, I suspect, be one such consequence. And it may be not the only one. Shortly after this "delayed infection" idea was proposed for leukaemia, essentially the same idea, the *hygiene hypothesis*, was suggested for the epidemic of allergies and type I diabetes, multiple sclerosis and certain other autoimmune diseases of young people, all of which appear to be afflictions of affluent and modern societies. The highest risk for all these problems is in the same region — Scandinavia. This really is an idea that I find irresistible, that we have a slew of modern illnesses that are the paradoxical consequence of progress. And that this is due to a mismatch between our past evolutionary programming (of the immune system) and our current lifestyles. Interesting maybe, and plausible, but is it right?

Scientific explanations often start out as no more than hunches, then there will be a search for supportive evidence. Definite proof can be hard to find and so it has proven to be though we are certainly much closer than we were 20 years ago. If the idea is that it's not a specific virus that causes leukaemia but actually an aberrant, dysregulated immune system somehow stressing the bone marrow and triggering preexistent leukaemia cells spawned before birth, how can this be either endorsed or disproved? It isn't at all easy to pose this question decisively, especially as we have had no idea what sorts of infections might be important. One could guess, from our evolutionary selection viewpoint, mycobacteria (related to those causing tuberculosis) or even common bacterial or viral respiratory infections might be involved, but we really don't know. The idea itself has attracted considerable international and media attention, in part, I suspect because of the dearth of plausible alternative explanations of the causes of childhood leukaemia. But also maybe because it smells of common sense, or grandma's wisdom: "a little bit of dirt does you good"?

One test we thought might prove informative was formulated as part of a very large and expensive (£15 million plus) nationwide study of children with leukaemia initiated around 1990 in the UK and which epidemiologists, clinicians and biologists, for the first time, got their heads together on this question. A parallel study, replicating the UK effort, was set up some years later in California. Over 1500 children with ALL were studied along with AML, other cancers and, for comparison, 4000 or so normal healthy children. We had a broad brief to look at all possible causes of leukaemia that had been of public concern, including infection, ionising radiation, non-ionising radiation from electromagnetic fields (EMF) (power lines, in house wiring, etc.), chemicals and genetic, inherited factors. Ten years later, the first results emerged. Ionising radiation and EMF appeared to have a minor, if any, role contrary to what some scientists and environmentalists believed, and still believe. This remains a highly contentious and unresolved issue. And one can understand why some parents, including Delena Fernandes and her husband, as she explains (Chapter 6), still focus on what must seem to them an obvious and local hazardous exposure. We cannot say that no cases of childhood leukaemia are ever caused by such radiation exposures, only that the evidence suggests that most are not. The most striking and positive data to emerge from both the UK and Californian studies were that infants who attended playgroups or crèches in the first year of life and had multiple contacts with other children had a reduced risk of childhood ALL. Other studies had similarly shown they had a reduced risk of allergies and type I diabetes. Playgroups are well recognised as hotbeds of infection spread and so the paradox was that somehow infection early in life appears to protect against ALL. But this is exactly what the hypothesis predicted. The results look convincing.

Home and dry? Not quite. Epidemiology is a very complex art form and there are always caveats and contradictory data. The detailed arguments do not matter here. It is suffice to say that more direct evidence is required. So, the hunt goes on. As it happens, we have recently uncovered, in the laboratory, a specific biochemical mechanism in which a hormonal product of a very active immune system can selectively stimulate the outgrowth of preleukaemic clones of cells. This certainly endorses the credibility of the aberrant immune response explanation. Now other doors have been opened up by technological innovation, with the human genome project in particular. It is now possible, in a way that was inconceivable 20 years ago, to scrutinise the entire human DNA code for variations in genes between individuals that might increase or decrease susceptibility to disease. This is already paying rich dividends in breast and colon cancers and certain autoimmune diseases. Needless to say, the prospect of being able to identify who is most at risk of what disease is far-reaching. For childhood leukaemia, the definitive, or what I hope will be the definitive, study is being planned just now as I write. The anticipation here is that the DNA variations that confer susceptibility will include genes that encode components of the immune system, or if not, then other functions that signify relevant exposures. For example, if variations in genes that encode enzymes that detoxify certain classes of toxic environmental chemicals turn out to be important, then this would automatically finger the corresponding chemicals as prime suspects. We will just have to wait and see.

I remain, as always, naïvely optimistic that there will be a clear outcome. But if it's not what I suspect, then here's the unwritten rule of scientific life: you have to be prepared to jettison your pet ideas and move on. If I'm right, on the other hand, then the prospect would be for some kind of prophylactic vaccine given to all infants that would prevent a substantial fraction, though not all, of childhood leukaemia. Now, that's a hope worth holding on to.

Journey's End?

Scientific research, and the knowledge base it provides constantly evolves. By the time this book is published, there will be some new insights into the biology of childhood leukaemia. Just in the past few years, we have learnt that leukaemic cell clones (and those of cancer in general) are organised in a kind of cellular hierarchy with a very small fraction ($< 1\%$) of primitive founder or stem cells sustaining the disease. This is a critical new insight since these cells, rather than the bulk disease, are the focus of evolutionary changes in the clone over time and must be the essential target for therapeutic elimination. We now see a different and more focussed target (see Epilogue below for a twin 'twist in the tale'). The chase never ends but after thirty or so years of travel in the landscape of childhood leukaemia, it's timely to reflect on where I, and fellow white-coated voyagers, are on the map? Well, we are one heck of a distance from the starting point for sure. But, to be realistic, the ultimate objective is still, tantalisingly, some way off. And, indeed, will remain so as long as some children like Georgie, whose story is told by her mum, Nicola, in Chapter 5 still succumb to their leukaemia. Or while others suffer long term side effects of the treatment and the causes are not ambiguously nailed as avoidable or preventable exposures. But the grounds for optimism are very tangible. We started off this journey in a fog, but, equipped with the extraordinarily illuminating tools of molecular biology and genetics, we can now see what paths to take. There will be false turns, setbacks and surprises, as always in science, but the prospects for more specific targeted and minimally toxic therapy are not just pipe dreams. No magic bullet, no quick fix but an eventual resolution nonetheless. And I have no doubt also that, before long, causation will no longer be a mystery to befuddle scientists, physicians, parents and patients, alike.

Epilogue: A Tale of Two Twins

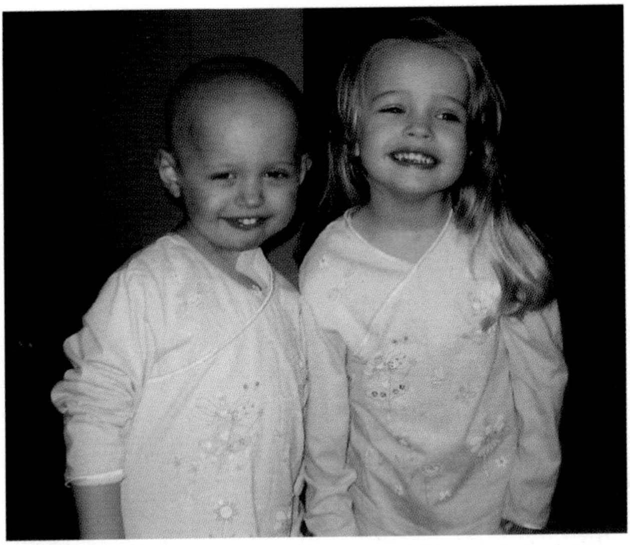

Fig. 14. Twins, Olivia and Isabella Murphy. (with permission of parents)

The Murphy family live just outside London. In 2003, Sarah gave birth to identical twin girls, Olivia and Isabella. As infants and toddlers, their development and general health were perfectly normal. But in 2005, aged 2½, Olivia was diagnosed with ALL. This was, to say the very least, bad news, but the mitigating fact was that Olivia's ALL was of the very good prognosis subtype — B cell precursor (common) ALL with the *TEL-AML1* fusion gene. She underwent the now standard two year regime of combination chemotherapy, and at the time of writing (April 2008), she is off treatment, in complete remission, and has an excellent chance of complete recovery. But alas, things are not that simple. Firstly, during her therapy, Olivia developed an attack of shingles (chicken pox) and as a consequence, she lost the sight in one eye. This was almost certainly a consequence of the immunosuppressive impact of the drugs given to combat the leukaemia — a tragic but not uncommon consequence of "collateral" damage of non-specific or toxic, drugs. This understandably caused the parents considerable distress. The parents were interviewed as part of a series of TV films on childhood leukaemia made by the company Mentorn and shown on BBC1 in July 2007. In the film, Dad, Jason, recalled how Olivia's loss of sight had shocked and upset him almost as much as the leukaemia itself. He and his wife were terrified that she might be left blind if the other eye also succumbed, which, fortunately, it has not.

Jason and Sarah also vividly recalled another aspect of their emotional engagement with leukaemia that is unique to their situation as the parents of twins and where one twin has leukaemia and the other does not. The twins are genetically identical and before Olivia developed ALL, they looked indistinguishable to anyone but the parents. As the parents watched Olivia transit through all the traumas and difficulties of treatment, they inevitably looked at Olivia's appearance in comparison with how she should and would, without ALL and chemotherapy, have looked like — just like her twin sister. Aside from the temporary loss of her hair, Olivia's growth slowed down such that she was smaller in size than Isabella and, as the parents reflected, she could be taken for her younger sister. Now, off treatment, Olivia's hair has grown back. Curiously, it is a somewhat different colour and more curly than before. The girls do look equally healthy and lovely now.

But then the parents have had another challenge to face. As Isabella is Olivia's identical twin sister, what about her risk of developing ALL? This very worrying question will inevitably occur to any parents in this situation and they will certainly ask their doctor about it. In the relatively recent past, some parents have been misinformed by doctors who obviously had the children's best interest at heart but were uncertain about the underlying biology. I know of contrasting situations where the parents have in one case been told words to the effect that "it's inevitable the second twin will get leukaemia", to another where the paediatrician said the chance was "less than one in a million". Both are way off the mark. The first thing that parents should be told is that there is a significantly increased risk but this has little or nothing to do with coinheritance of some "susceptibility" gene by the twins and that, by the same token, any other sibling would have no or very little risk inherited.

When Olivia was diagnosed and with the help of her physician Dr Philip Ancliff at Great Ormond Street Hospital in London, we were able to discuss the actual risk involved and what might be done about it. We know from our longstanding studies that the risk of a "double diagnosis" comes from the sharing of a single placenta in the womb and the consequent sharing of blood. Olivia and Isabella did have a single placenta (some 40 percent of identical twins do not). Based on the available data on concordance of disease in twins with ALL of the common subtype, we calculated that at the time Olivia was diagnosed, the risk to her healthy twin sister Isabella was approximately 10 percent or one in ten. This is of course significantly increased (by 200 times) from the standard risk of any child of one in 2000 but there was still a 90 percent or so probability that Isabella would *not* develop ALL; good or bad odds depending on how you look at it (and whether you're a parent or an observer!). As was detailed earlier in this chapter, ALL begins with one mutant cell arising in the developing baby in the womb but only emerges as a clinical disease if a second, independent mutation arises in the same cell clone within the following few years. The chances are stacked against the second "hit" occurring at all such that in 90 percent of identical twin pairs, when one does have the second "hit" and hence ALL, the other will not. Sarah and Jason were remarkably astute in readily comprehending this complexity, to the point that Sarah made a very perceptive observation. This was that although Olivia but not Isabella had ALL, the first hit generating the leukaemic clone could have happened in Isabella. This is absolutely correct as a possibility but there is no way of knowing.

The advice given to the parents in this case was that it would be prudent to serially monitor Isabella's blood for signs of ALL. If the results were consistently negative, then this would be reassuring but if the one in ten chance came up, then at least the disease would be caught very early and the prospects for cure would be very high. This wasn't an easy call for Sarah and Jason. Isabella would have to have blood taken regularly, not a happy prospect for any child or her parents and, additionally, they would, in effect, be in constant anticipation of a possible positive result. Nevertheless, they opted for this course. So, for the past three years, every four to six weeks Isabella has provided a blood sample that has been sent across London from Great Ormond Street Hospital to my laboratory. What we have found has taught us a great deal about the biology of ALL so that the family have made a real contribution to our understanding and deserve our gratitude. What we had long anticipated from our previous twin studies, coupled with the neonatal blood spots, was that Isabella would have, in her blood, what we call the "pre-leukaemic" cell clone. These are cells that are shared by the twins and have "hit 1" mutation, which in Olivia's case, was the common fusion gene called *TEL-AML1*. Two further predictions were as follows. First, that these cells, in Isabella, should only be present at the low level we observed before in newborn cord blood — which would be around one per every 1000 normal lymphocytes. This would be millions-fold less than present in Olivia's blood at diagnosis. And, second, that these rare cells, though harbouring malignant potential, would lack the additional mutational gene changes present at diagnosis in Olivia's ALL cells. This is exactly what was found in the serial blood samples of Isabella's blood. From the purely academic perspective, this has given us a unique insight. It also provided us with a source of pre-malignant ALL cells that we are using for further research so that we could determine their inherent risk of evolving to full blown ALL. From the family's perspective, we could reassure them that the presence of such cells, given the twin context, was as anticipated (but previously unproven) and that these pre-leukaemic cells have remained silent, docile, and at the same very low level. So what now? Our twin data set suggest that the 10 percent risk declines with age and will be very low by the time Isabella is a teenager. Most twins develop ALL within one or two years of each other, and in the many twin pairs we have studied, only one has developed ALL much later (age 14, nine years after her sister).

The Murphy twins offered us another unique opportunity. They provided a chance to interrogate different stages of the leukaemic process; to, in effect, watch a process unfolding that is normally invisible. In collaboration with a colleague, Professor Tariq Enver and his team in Oxford, we were able to identify, for the first time, in Isabella, the rare stem cells that drive and sustain the pre-leukaemic phase and which, in Olivia's case, evolved to stem cells generating florid or clinical leukaemia. This stem cell evolutionary process we could show was associated with the acquisition, in Olivia's stem cells (but not in Isabella's), of additional genetic mutations. Stem cells in leukaemia, and other cancers, are the most critical cellular component of the disease. These relatively rare cells continuously spawn large numbers of clonal progeny cells (which cause the pathology), they are the focus for further malignant evolution by mutation and, most importantly, the cells that the therapy has to silence or eliminate. Having a handle on these cells in childhood leukaemia is a very significant advance.

We published these exciting studies in the journal *Science* at the beginning of 2008. These attracted extensive media coverage in the UK and abroad. Why was this so? We would like to think that the science was innovative and certainly there is a great deal of public interest in stem cells. But, undoubtedly, what really "sold" the story was the role played by two rather special little girls.

Acknowledgements

The author wishes to express his gratitude for those funding bodies and organisations that have generously supported his research over many years. These include The Imperial Cancer Research Fund (now part of CR-UK), The Institute of Cancer Research (London), The Kay Kendall Leukaemia Fund (UK) and the Leukaemia Research Fund (UK). Many thanks also to the many colleagues who have been fellow travellers and wonderful companions on this journey.

General References

1. Greaves M, The causation of childhood leukaemia: a paradox of progress? *Discov Med*, **6**: 24–28, 2006.
2. Greaves M, *Cancer. The Evolutionary Legacy*, Oxford University Press, Oxford, 2000. *This book explains how evolution has bequeathed vulnerability to cancer and other diseases.*
3. Greaves M, Childhood leukaemia, *Br Med J*, **324**: 283–287, 2002.

Technical References

1. Greaves MF, Wiemels J, Origins of chromosome translocations in childhood leukaemia, *Nat Rev Cancer*, **3**: 639–649, 2003.
2. Greaves MF, Maia AT, Wiemels JL, Ford AM, Leukaemia in twins: lessons in natural history, *Blood*, **102**: 2321–2333, 2003.
3. Greaves M, Infection, immune responses and the aetiology of childhood leukaemia, *Nat Rev Cancer*, **6**: 193–203, 2006.

A CHILD PSYCHOLOGIST'S JOURNEY

Jeanette van Dongen-Melman

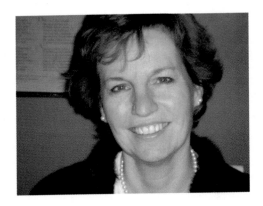

A CHILD PSYCHOLOGIST'S JOURNEY

Jeanette van Dongen-Melman

People often ask me, "How can you work with children who have leukaemia? It must be difficult."

My reply is, "Actually, it isn't. It is wonderful to work with them. Children with leukaemia and their parents are just ordinary people like you and me. They show how strong and resilient one can be when one is faced with hardship. They also teach you about life, its good and bad things, how to accept and overcome misfortune and that it is possible to undergo great difficulties and survive emotionally. Most of them want to fight the disease, and consequently, learn to accept the suffering that accompanies it. What I learn from them is to be brave, to be happy with what you've got, to celebrate today and not wait until tomorrow."

I also reply with, "Yes it is, it is very difficult to work with children with leukaemia. It is gruesome to see them suffering everyday. It touches your heart time and again when you see their small, bleak faces, holding their favourite stuffed animal that is worn out from being cuddled in their thin arms while they walk with their uncertain, wobbly gait on their frail legs to the doctor for yet another medical examination, a puncture or a course of chemotherapy. I can only treat these children because they are not my own. It hurts to see their thin, fragile bodies, to watch them suffer, and to see them confronted with situations no child should face."

Then I tell them the story of an 8-year-old boy with leukaemia who came to my office for psychological testing. It was a beautiful sunny summer morning. While he was filling in a questionnaire, I offered to get him a glass of lemonade. He liked that. When I returned, the following picture became etched in my memory: a child working steadfast with pencil in hand, and behind him, sunshine poured through the window on the desk where he was working. On that brightly lit desk, I noticed a dark spot, a tuft of neatly combed hair. He looked up from his work as I entered the room and explained in an apologetic tone: "It was so hot; I had to take off my wig." I realized that while I was away fetching his lemonade, he must have been contemplating such questions as, "Shall I take off my wig or not? How will she react when she sees I'm bald? If I take it off, should I say something or not? What should I say?" The fact that these children have to spend time contemplating such things instead of mulling about whether they should go out to play with friends or stay at home on the computer is so unfair.

Moreover, it is very unfair to their parents. Their worst nightmare seems to be coming true: losing their child. It's very moving when you see the love and care parents provide their children. I read the anxiety and concern on their faces, whereas at the same time, they maintain a brave and optimistic attitude. I see their concern in letting their children move about by themselves while at the same time trying to be there exactly when their children need support. I wonder how it is possible for parents to accept this ordeal, how they can go on with life and their additional responsibilities to their other children, to their work and household chores while living with the constant threat of losing their child. In addition, they have to make choices for an uncertain future and to consent to begin treatment. How can they go along with treatment when they do not know what the rigors and consequences of treatment are? What if the harsh treatment doesn't work and the child dies or finishes treatment and has serious long-term side effects? What if their child is drastically changed because of the treatment? With these uncertainties and questions in the parents' minds, I started my PhD thesis with the following quotation from a television film in which a psychotherapist treats a traumatised patient named Sybil.

> *One day Dr Wilbur asked Sybil:*
> *"How do you prepare yourself for the misfortunes in your life?"*
> *"You never are prepared for catastrophes," replied Sybil, "They just happen;*
> *and that is what makes you prepared."*[a]

In this chapter, I will depict the psychological issues involved in childhood leukaemia. The psychological impact of childhood leukaemia is related directly to its treatment options, the course of the disease, and its prognosis. I will first provide a brief overview of these issues to serve as background information. Then I will address the many psychological difficulties children with leukaemia and their families face during treatment and beyond.

The Start of the Journey

I began working with children with leukaemia in 1982 when cure rates rose and hopes were high that if a child was diagnosed with leukaemia, he or she could survive the disease. It was not long before that when leukaemia was almost inevitably fatal. Before the late 1960s and early 1970s, less than 20 percent of the children survived leukaemia for more than two years. Consequently, the child with leukaemia was treated as a dying child from diagnosis onwards. As Don Pinkel describes in his chapter, the survival rates increased as a result of the combined application of radiotherapy and chemotherapy. Further improvement was achieved by more aggressive and intensive treatment protocols, and in the 1980s, 60 to 70 percent of the children survived their disease for more than five years. In less than 20 years, a spectacular improvement of the survival rates for children with leukaemia was accomplished. With contemporary treatment protocols, as many as 75 to 85 percent of these children survive.

[a]From *Sybil*, directed by Daniel Petri, USA (1976).

Along with the progress in medical treatment, childhood leukaemia changed from an acute fatal illness, into a chronic life-threatening disease but with a real chance for cure. Instead of adapting to the imminence of death, the psychological focus shifted on living with leukaemia and planning for an uncertain future. Therefore, if children had a real chance of survival, it was important that they should be able to go on with their lives once they were cured. Because a child's development does not stop with a diagnosis of leukaemia, the objective became the maintenance of as many aspects of normal day-to-day functioning as possible. Treating children with leukaemia as "normally" as possible in every aspect of their life became a key objective, which also implies that the child should stay in his or her natural environment, that is to say, at home, as much as possible during treatment. This resulted in shortened hospital stays and the implementation of treatment on an outpatient basis. To achieve this goal, parents became a part of the healthcare team and were taught to give the necessary care and medication to their child at home.

Normal life and planning for a child's future also means going to school and having interactions with peers. Just as parents needed to be taught that their child had a real chance to live on, teachers now had to be informed about the improved prognosis. An important prejudice that had to be dispelled was their fear that the child could suddenly die in their classroom. After removing uncertainties about the disease and informing teachers about the emotional needs of these children, emphasising that they need to be dealt with in the same manner as any other child, they were welcomed back into the classroom. This is a very anxious time for parents because the treatment of leukaemia suppresses the child's immune system and therefore otherwise innocuous or mild infectious diseases in healthy children such as chicken pox can be fatal. Nevertheless, most parents were brave and let their child go to school and take part in outdoor activities while taking all sorts of precautions. Others kept their child at home as much as possible, thereby isolating the child for the length of the treatment which at that time lasted two years. Understandably, parents felt confronted with the choice between life and death on the one hand and a normal development on the other.

As more and more children survived their disease, however, the costs of cure gradually became apparent. The rigorous treatment necessary to eradicate leukaemic cells also affects normal cells. An increasing number of studies appeared in the literature that reported late medical side effects, such as disorders in growth and puberty, neuropsychological deficits including a decline in IQ and learning difficulties, dysfunction of the heart, lungs and kidneys and secondary malignancies. Some side effects also have cosmetic implications. Dental damage, problems with hair growth, and scarring, facial deformities, stunted growth, and obesity all have a direct effect on the child's appearance. An understanding that disease-free survival is not identical to cure, led to a new view about "being cured". In his influential book, *The truly cured child*,[b] Jan Van Eys, a paediatric oncologist, explained in 1977 that disease-free survival is not synonymous with cure, but should extend to the quality of survival. Consequently, the psychological and social consequences of childhood leukaemia also need to be taken into account when treating a child with leukaemia.

In that time that warranted an optimistic view on survival, there was so much emphasis on living with leukaemia during active treatment, that the fatal nature of leukaemia became blurred. As long as childhood leukaemia is not a completely curable disease, the life-threatening aspect of the disease remains present. Children and parents must learn how to live with the disease as well as having to prepare for the possibility that the child might die. The fact that a child might die of leukaemia is the most significant issue concerning leukaemia for parents. The turmoil resulting from a diagnosis of leukaemia, still today, is a direct and justifiable reaction to this threat. Whereas adults immediately associate leukaemia with death, this is

[b]Van Eys J (ed). *The Truly Cured Child.* Baltimore MD, University Park Press, 1977.

less obvious to a child. Therefore, it is important to have insight into how children become aware of the seriousness of their leukaemia.

Becoming Aware of the Life-Threatening Nature of Leukaemia is a Process

Before I started working with children with leukaemia, one of the leading themes in psychology was whether or not the children should be told about their diagnosis of leukaemia. Proponents of the protective approach based their arguments on the existing literature of a child's intellectual understanding of death. Before the age of 10, children have immature notions about death, and thus could not be afraid of death unless they are told of the potentially fatal prognosis. Consequently, shielding children from the diagnosis was the preferred option. In addition, it was observed that children seldom ask questions about their illness, which was interpreted as a lack of concern about the disease on the part of the child. This view was challenged; claiming that if a child is shielded from the diagnosis, his unrealistic fantasies are fed, which causes an increase of anxiety, withdrawn behaviour and depressive symptoms. Furthermore, it was argued that children will not ask any further questions when they observe how upset their parents become by these questions. Due to the misreading of the children's awareness of the seriousness of their disease, the adults also remain silent. To avoid this situation of blocked communication, it was advised to inform the children about the diagnosis and to keep communication open about their concerns. In addition to the arguments as to why children should be informed about their disease and treatment, the improved prognosis of childhood leukaemia clearly sped up this change in approach and the issue as to whether or not the children should be told about their leukaemia diagnosis was resolved in favor of disclosing it to them.

With that said, how do you tell young children about their diagnosis of leukaemia? This is particularly relevant for leukaemia for which half of the children with it are diagnosed before the age of five. The child's understanding of the life-threatening aspect of leukaemia depends on its cognitive age. In contrast to adults, a child will not immediately grasp the potentially fatal prognosis, but will only become aware of the seriousness of the disease gradually. The crucial issue here is the child's *experience* with the disease.

Children's first experience with leukaemia is that they are ill. They will find out that they are ill by feeling unwell; a visit to the doctor, a worried look on the parent's face with tears in their eyes, parents coming home from work at unusual times, or muffled conversations that are followed by an unexpected sudden rush to the hospital without any preparation. Being at the hospital is an overwhelming experience for children. They are confronted with an unknown environment and unknown people; *"The bed in the hospital is different from the one you have at home and you see all kind of strange children lying around you."*[c] There is also a change in daily rhythm; *"You are not allowed to go to your own school and you don't see your friends anymore."* However, the separation from their parents makes the deepest impression and children experience great anxiety when parents leave the hospital (Fig. 15).

> *"I always started to cry when my parents left the hospital."*
>
> *"It's actually strange that you have to stay in the hospital when your parents leave, because you belong to your parents. And when they go away and come back and still leave you behind, that's strange. It feels as if you don't belong to them anymore."*
>
> *"I was afraid they (parents) left me alone."*
>
> *"I always worry if my parents will return to me again."*

Parents are bewildered and shocked when they learn about the diagnosis: *"When your child is in danger of dying, it really drives you crazy. Believe me, you go out of your mind. It's the end of your world. Your whole house comes crashing down."* In a situation which is so different than it used to be, children look to their parents in order to assess their new situation. As a result, the parents' reaction to the

---

[c]All quotations are derived from clinical interviews by the author with patients, their parents and siblings.

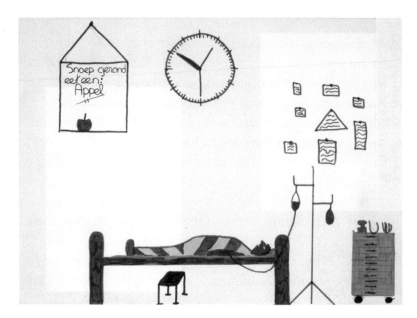

Fig. 15.   Vincent's drawing. The child is alone in the hospital receiving treatment. While the chemotherapy is dripping into his body, he watches the big clock and counts the seconds until his parents are coming to visit him. Vincent is ten years old.

diagnosis of leukaemia gives children very important cues about their situation and they learn about their disease by watching their parent's distress.

> *"My father almost never cries. When he did, it must have been very serious."*
>
> *"My mother always walked out into the hallway with a handkerchief."*
>
> *"...and my mother, all that crying."*
>
> *"They (parents) were not happy anymore and then I started to think, 'hey, what's going on here'?"*

The emotional climate in a child's life changes with the diagnosis of leukaemia. This not only occurs with the parents and other immediate family members, but also with extended family members like grandparents and other relatives. Furthermore, friends, school teachers, neighbours and acquaintances also approach the child differently now that they know that the child is ill. Children are quite capable of discerning these subtle changes.

Another source of information for the children about the seriousness of their disease is the nature of the treatment they receive. The treatment for leukaemia is long and intensive. This requires frequent hospital visits for check-ups and therapy. The treatment period is two years according to contemporary protocols. Time goes by very slowly for children, so it is important to realise that they have a different perception of time than adults do. Consequently, it's impossible for a child to comprehend the length of treatment. In their perception, it goes on forever.

> *"My disease lasted quite long, very long, actually!"*

They may start to wonder why they still have not been cured. In the meantime, the child has to undergo frequent medical procedures such as bone marrow aspirations, lumbar and venous punctures, injections or infusions of chemotherapeutic agents that are painful and distressing for the child. This signals to the child that something serious is going on.

> *"I didn't want to go to the bone marrow punctures. I found them gruesome. Especially the last one when the doctor used a needle that went right through my spine. That hurts a lot. And when we drove away from the hospital, it felt as if all those needles were still stuck in my spine."*

Often, the child feels worse because of the treatment.

> *"They draw way too much blood out of me, way too much; soon I won't live anymore."*
> *"All these punctures are gonna break my bones."*

The treatment for leukaemia is continued at home and the child is confronted with taking medications, a special diet, sufficient fluid intake, and mouth care, along with all the other caretaking procedures on a daily basis. Many children have difficulties in swallowing the amount of pills, as one child recalls, *"You get mad and crazy from all these medicines, sometimes you have to vomit and that makes you even more crazy!"*

Chemotherapy is the first choice in treating childhood leukaemia but has a number of unwanted side effects, including

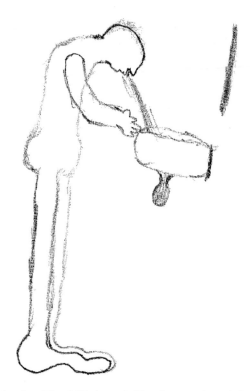

Fig. 16.   Mark's drawing. The child almost bald, only some down left, shows how unwell and miserable he is from the chemotherapy. Mark is thirteen years old.

vomiting, allergic reactions, mouth ulcers, loss of hair, weight gain and weight loss. For children, it is strange that medications that are supposed to cure you and make you feel better, in fact, make you feel worse.

> *"These medicines, all they do is just make me more sick."*

For children, it is difficult to understand that treatment can in fact make them feel worse (Fig. 16). How children feel is an important source of information for them about the seriousness of their disease. Many children feel that their physical condition is different than it was before the disease. If a child feels well and encounters a few difficulties from the disease, a child will become hopeful that the disease will eventually disappear. However, when children experience complications, feel ill, tired and weak, or when they relapse and treatment has to be implemented again, they may wonder if cure is an option. In fact, the children's physical condition is a signal for them that indicates how seriously ill they are.

The clearly visible side effects that anyone can notice affect children very much, because they are a constant reminder that they are different from their peers. The loss of hair is especially hard for children, as Janine recalls in Chapter 6.

> *"They called me names like 'baldy' and then I wore a cap, but then they tear my cap off."*

The reactions of adults and peers to the visible side effects are a constant source of fear and worry for the child. They constantly challenge the child's social skills, which are in fact, only in development at this time in their lives and not fully equipped to deal with these extra difficult situations. In addition, they may be confronted with reactions about the life threatening nature of their disease, as a child describes, *"A classmate asked if I was going to die because he was told by his mother that I had leukaemia and was going to die."* Most children feel uncertain and unable to cope when they are confronted with these sensitive questions about their disease; their absences from school; being teased about their physical appearance and being rebuffed in social interaction. Furthermore, they have to be constantly alert, because they never know when someone will make an unexpected move or when a difficult situation is to be expected. As a result, children with leukaemia derive less pleasure from the interaction with their peers and thus distance themselves from these situations. Although the direct side effects disappear once treatment is over, most children find them horrifying.

Dealing with Emotions Resulting from Leukaemia

Many parents wish to know what is going on in their child's mind in order to support them. As a result, parents ask their children questions to gain insight into their inner world. However, often, children aren't able to respond to these questions easily because they cannot put their experiences and emotions into words.

> *"I wanted to tell them so, but I just couldn't."*
>
> *"I wanted to tell them once, but my parents were just about to go home and then I couldn't explain it."*

Moreover, children have numerous additional reasons for not telling what burdens them. For instance, they fear that others are not likely to respond or will respond negatively:

> *"I could have asked the doctor about my disease, but I didn't, for he won't tell you right away, because he will ask your parents first whether you're allowed to know the diagnosis."*
>
> *"I just don't let on about things. I just don't let on about a lot of things, because otherwise, they will find me stupid or something and then they'd call me 'softie' or say something like 'you're no match. You just can't take anything.'"*

Besides, children may expect negative consequences resulting from open communication and try to avoid these by keeping their worries to themselves.

> *"Suppose I let them know I was worried, and then they surely would have kept me longer in the hospital."*
>
> *"I held it (negative feelings) all to myself, because if I let it out, you know, I thought my parents will get mad at me."*
>
> *".. my mother tells me, 'you can always talk to me', but I just don't dare. I'm afraid that if I do, they will leave me, and all I want to is to stay with my parents."*

In addition, children don't want to show their emotions in order to keep their own emotional balance.

> *"It is best for you if you just don't have to talk about it, otherwise I start crying."*
>
> *"I never want to talk about it, because there's always something that's mentioned that I don't like."*

Another issue the child encounters in expressing the concerns related to leukaemia, is that children love their parents above all and don't want them be upset.

*"If I would talk to them, then everything at home is in a state of uproar,
then my mother will start worrying again."*
"My mother always starts to cry."

Children wish to help their parents when they withhold their concerns about their disease. Caring for family members includes that parents care for their children, but children also care for their parents. This latter aspect is often overlooked in paediatric psychology; however, in the literature on family therapy, these mutual caring processes are an essential ingredient of defining a family as such. In addition, when children notice that their parents become upset, they also become upset. Thus, in keeping worries and feelings to themselves, children care for their parents **and** for their own emotional wellbeing.

Misconceptions about Dealing with Emotions

There are some common notions about dealing with emotions that seriously hamper the child's coping process. The general idea is that in order to reduce emotions, they should be expressed, and if the individual does not, this is considered a sign of "bad" coping. If emotions are not released, they will crop up and hence hinder the individual's well being. Moreover, emotions may even increase over time, resulting in a more intense outburst later on. However, the question is whether coping processes can be sped up and worked on in advance, like with homework or chores. Coping is performing emotional labour and that needs time. A natural, normal coping process consists of a continuous swing between expressing emotions and suppressing them (note that suppression is not the same as denial). Working through emotions costs so much energy that emotionally tranquil periods are necessary to regain energy in order to confront a painful emotion once again. Distraction from the illness by focusing on other aspects in life is a way of doing so. Coping is balancing between focusing on disease-related issues and focusing on issues not related to the disease. My worry is that the well-intended emphasis on open communication might push the children too hard to express their feelings, thereby interfering with and disturbing the delicate balance between confrontation and avoidance. Research shows that the suppression of emotions as such is not related to maladjustment, and that too much expression of emotions has adverse effects. Therefore, all those involved in supporting the child with leukaemia, parents, teachers, family, friends and the healthcare team should respect the natural coping process of children and approach them in a way that fits in with their strategies of dealing with the disease.

Reading the Child's Behaviour and Responding to It

It may help parents to know that many children are aware of their delicate situation, even if they don't express it in ways that are clear to us as adults. To state it even more boldly, children just cannot make it clear in ways we as adults *want* them to. We rely almost exclusively on language, probably for our own convenience, and probably because we ourselves are uncertain what the child may know about leukaemia. We often forget that language is just one method of communication. Even when language is used, only about 30 percent of what we wish to express is communicated by words, whereas 70 percent of the message is conveyed by non-verbal language, such as tone, facial expression, posture and behaviour. We humans have a whole range of behaviour at our disposal with which we can communicate. Because we strongly focus on language, we forget the other ways of expression that are often natural for a child in development. I recall the worry of a mother that her child was not coping well because he did not talk about his disease, while at the same time she mentioned that her child was drawing and playing out scenes from the hospital. Children treated for leukaemia know that there is or has been something terribly wrong with them. In my view, it is *our problem* that we have difficulty in *reading their behaviour*. In helping the children to cope with their illness, it is not a question of talking with them, but of reading their behaviour, and consequently, responding to it. T. Gordon's book, "*Parent Effectiveness Training*" explains this process, as does the parents' booklet, *All's well that ends well?* (see general references).

Children with leukaemia can cope with the many negative emotions evolving from the threat of death and the rigors of treatment when they feel loved by their parents and feel that they will not be left alone with their worries, unspoken fears and questions. In my experience, the saddest children were those who felt alone and/or were left alone with their unpleasant feelings. Negative emotions such as sadness, pain, worries, fear, anger, jealousy and hopelessness are bearable for a child if they are recognized and can be shared.

Parents of Children with Leukaemia: Where do We Go from Here?

How can you support your child when you've just learned that your child has leukaemia? Children are the most precious things in life for parents. They love them more than they love themselves; hence, to lose their child is the worst that could possibly happen to parents.

> *"When I heard that Marion had leukaemia, I thought 'this is the end', nothing is sacred in life anymore."*
>
> *"The only thing there is, is my kid, and there's nothing else but fear, pure fear."*

Upon hearing the diagnosis, parents want to know whether treatment will cure the disease.

> *"The doctors wanted to start treatment, in fact, a whole lot of treatment. That worried me to the utmost because I wasn't sure if treatment made sense. I wanted to know if he had a chance. Should you start treatment? Should my child be under medical treatment for such a long time, just so that when it's all over we could say, 'at least we tried all we could and it's a pity that we lost him?' Or do you have to say, 'he has a fair chance of surviving, say 50 percent.' Then you think, 'For God's sake, just get started!'*

However, the contemporary 80 percent chance of survival is tricky. It is a figure that tells nothing about how a statistical risk is perceived and weighed. In the perception and assessment of risks, the mechanisms outside the realm of mathematics operate. Parents want to know the chances for *their* child and a survival figure *per se* tells nothing about their specific situation. Therefore, even if the chance for cure is high, the life threatening aspect of the disease still stands out. In addition, the interpretation of chances is dependent on the parents' own experience with their child's disease:

> "I don't think we were really afraid, at least not in the beginning. It started when he came home from the hospital and fell so ill."

> "When she was diagnosed, for me, it was just the end; it was all over because she was so ill. There was no life in her at all. And still in August, after five months in the hospital, she came home for the very first time, she was so ill that my husband and I said to each other, 'She won't make it to Christmas'."

Another powerful illustration of the psychological mechanisms involved in risk assessment is that even though fathers and mothers receive the same prognostic information and have similar experiences with their child's illness, they can have different perceptions about the chance for survival:

> Mother: "The one thing I could think of was: 'He is going to die'."
> Father: "I have never ever thought about that, not for one moment."
> Mother: "I did, I didn't know how, where or when, but I did know he was going to die."

As a result of the outcome of weighing risks at diagnosis, parents range on a continuum from "no hope" to "extreme hope." This perspective might change during the course of treatment. If the child stays alive, most parents flip from a death perspective to a survival perspective. Mothers especially seem to take on an intense and strong survival perspective directly after hearing the diagnosis:

> "The moment the doctor told us he has leukaemia, then pop, instantly you switch around, 'okay, so now I know and now, now we are going to fight. Yes it is really true, but we won't allow things to get out of hand, you see, we are just going to handle it all down to the minutest detail so the child won't die.'"

For parents, the diagnosis of leukaemia is an unexpected blow and many of them want to know how this could have happened, *"You keep asking yourself why he got ill. He's only three years old. He's never even done anything wrong, like smoking or drinking."* Parents may question themselves if they had done something wrong, or if they could have done something positively to have prevented the disease. For some parents, the unknown cause of leukaemia plays a role in refraining them from having future children, even though they had thought about having a bigger family, *"I was considering it, one or two, and when he was ill, then I knew it immediately, that's it, isn't it? Absolutely no more children, I don't want this to happen again."*

For parents, the child's treatment involves emotional as well as practical burdens in addition to the threat of losing their child. They must accept the rigors of treatment without any guarantee that it will cure the disease. They have to deal with informed consent procedures, hospitalizations, and repeated clinic visits; all these causing disruption from work routines and considerable financial expense. In addition, they have to watch their child suffer, which is unbearable:

> *"We feel so guilty, so terribly guilty about all that is happening to him, because you only wish one thing: for Gods sake, give me those punctures and hurt me, and stay away from my child."*

> *"And he looks you in the eye with an expression 'are you really letting this happen to me?' and there you are, helpless, and then you have to reassure yourself: yes, that is good for my child, that is best for my child; but I die inside, every time he's being hurt, I simply die."*

Parents feel helpless and want to make it up to their child. Their own emotional reaction to the rigours of treatment and the life threatening nature of the disease will influence their attitude about parenting. A natural reaction of parents is to indulge and protect their child. In this way, parenting becomes a useful and powerful tool, because it has short-term positive consequences both for the child and for themselves in view of the fact that parents' own negative emotions are also reduced when they see their child is less upset. Previously, indulging children was not encouraged because it was seen as spoiling, however, new insights show that indulging the child during treatment has direct positive effects as is beautifully described by Janine Fernandes, a patient herself, in her chapter. However, it all comes to balance and, in the long run, overprotection and overindulgence can jeopardize a child's development, as a parent explains.

> "On the one hand, you have a child that's ill and of course, you pamper a child who is ill. You are inclined to mollycoddle him. But, if this abnormal situation continues on and on as our situation did, which continued for weeks and months, then you should be aware that he shouldn't be mollycoddled forever. Just giving him 'no' for an answer sometimes was very important for him. In this way, he knew how far he could go. He needs that certainty, not only the certainty of our unconditional love, but also the certainty of having limits."

Day-to-day living with a child with leukaemia affects family life in numerous ways. Parents focus their time and energy on the ill child and logically give less attention to each other. In addition, a set of parents may have different perceptions on the outlook of the disease, and consequently, cope differently. As one set of parents explains:

> Mother: "The big difference between you and me was that for a long time you always saw things very negatively."
>
> Father: "For me it felt as if my child was already dead. You were like an iceberg, being optimistic about the outcome. I didn't understand that at all."
>
> Mother: "And I have no sympathy for people like you who just give up like that."
>
> Father: "And when I reacted differently than you did, I felt very alone; I really wanted to be together, but it didn't work. You're super lonely."

In this way, the leukaemia set limits to the expectation of standing together in stormy weather, which creates loneliness within a relationship and at times, great frictions. Despite the extra stresses on the relationship, couples seldom split up during the period of treatment.

Siblings: The Forgotten Children

Another change in family life is that parents tend to pay less attention to their other children. The ill child becomes the most important family member and the emotional atmosphere in the family is dependent on his or her physical and emotional well being. Siblings vividly notice this shift in attention:

"They (parents) just think about him, they are too worried about him, and so they don't think, 'perhaps she should have attention too', their mind is only on him."

"They (parents) are much more busy with my sister than with me, it's as if I don't belong anymore, as if I'm forgotten."

They feel they have a less important position within the family, and are not contributing to family happiness in a significant way anymore. The disruption siblings experience in the relationship with their parents is their major problem, especially when they have no reliable explanation to account for this change, considering children do not immediately grasp the implications of leukaemia. Talking with siblings gives a fascinating impression of how they perceive and interpret the diagnosis of leukaemia. In fact, it goes exactly along the same principles as with their ill sibling, namely according to their *own experiences*. However, because their experiences with the illness are so different from their ill sibling, their process of becoming aware of the diagnosis takes a different path.

Children have stereotypes about being ill and how to get better. They build their ideas about illness and health on their own experiences with illness. If one is ill, one has to stay in bed, occasionally a visit to or from the doctor is needed, and after a few days, one is better and carries on with life as before. When their ill sibling returns from the hospital or a doctor's visit, they expect the disease to be cured, as one sibling recalled, *"I thought, 'he's visiting the doctor, so he'll be better, because doctors always make you better'."* When the ill child is in the hospital, siblings often explain the prolonged absence in terms of daily activities known to them *"I thought she was playing at her friend's home"* or *"maybe he's staying with a friend or our grandparents."* In addition, siblings can misconstrue words used to refer to the illness or treatment process. For instance, the word *leukaemia* has the word 'leuk' in it, which in Dutch means 'fun'. *"In the beginning I thought, 'yes, leukaemia, when I heard that word, I thought you were "leuk" (funny/fun)'."*

Adults can unconsciously facilitate the misconception about the seriousness of the illness. Perhaps as a reaction to the appalling situation or to maintain hope for themselves, parents often emphasize the positive aspects in the hospital setting. They recall the pleasant and exciting moments for the ill child, *"They told me that there was a nice nurse which always played games with Paul and they had a lot of fun with squirting each other with water from syringes"*. They will talk about the playroom and play activities organized for children in the hospital, the many presents the child receives from visitors, the nice doctors and nurses that treat the child and the many facilities in the hospital such as having their own telephone, their own TV or computer in the room and choosing what to eat every day like they do for their birthday (Fig. 17). Furthermore, the sibling notices the differential treatment by their parents in favour of the ill child.

"All of my parents' attention went to my sister."

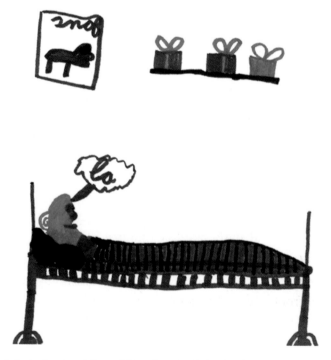

Fig. 17.   Arjan's drawing. Many siblings imagine being in the hospital as one big party. The patient receives many get well cards and lots of presents and as a result the patient, although bald, is happily singing in his bed. Arjan is eight years old.

> *"I knew that my parents were going to visit my sister in the hospital, but even so I thought they collected her and then went to visit somebody."*

As a result of these experiences and the child's age, a sibling has difficulties explaining the changes within the family and the special position of the ill child. Just as it is in the ill child, the siblings' own experience of the illness is an important source of information. In addition to what parents tell their children, the change in atmosphere at home and the anxiety and sorrow in their parents conveys important information about the seriousness of the disease.

> *"There were constant worries, there were always constant worries at home."*
>
> *"You're tense about what's going on and how it will end. You feel that it's not going well, that's for sure. That is what you are feeling even if you are very small."*

Visits to the hospital and being present during medical procedures help siblings to understand the seriousness of the disease. Also, the physical changes they see in their ill sibling have their effect:

> *"When I visited her, and I saw her with all those tubes and no hair, then I understood she was at the hospital, yeah, I just thought she was staying at her friend's house."*
>
> *"I hadn't seen her for such a long time, and I wanted to visit her so badly, and then I saw her..., I never wanted to see her ever again, what I saw hurt so much: she was totally bald,"*

The same hurdles that ill children have in expressing concerns and worries to their parents, also apply to their siblings. Most of all, they don't want their parents to be unhappy, *"Questions like, 'can he still die?' yeah, when you start to talk about it, they become very sad, and that's exactly what you don't want."* However, siblings are even more limited in expressing their emotions than their ill sibling because they are not confronted with anything tangible, such as hospitalizations, injections, therapy, and a potentially shortened life span, but rather, they have feelings of being left out, jealousy and resentment. Talking about feelings that are not related to a concrete situation is especially difficult for children *"Maybe I can let it show, but I actually don't know how to show it."* In addition, they may be reluctant to express these feelings because, at the same time, they notice how parents try to balance their attention and know very well that their ill sibling has had a more difficult time than they have had. "I just don't talk about it because then they'll say, 'you're not ill'."

If a Child Dies

The saddest time in paediatric oncology is when there is no longer any hope for cure. Often the child, the family and the healthcare team have traveled down a long road to cure, and it is very difficult when their efforts have not succeeded. During those moments, one questions whether the suffering of the child and family was worth the extra amount of time gained by treatment. When it is clear that further curative treatment is not an option, the last phase of the child's life starts. Most parents want to take their child home and give the child a "normal" life for as long as possible with less hospital visits and without painful medical procedures. In a last attempt to enjoy life and make up for the lost youth, children want to carry on as long as possible with their lives just like before their illness and often even want to go to school. For the child and family it is a very precious time where mutual love and care between child and parents prevails. As a child expressed, *"Just before I die, I'll tell my parents that when I am gone, they don't have to worry about me anymore, because I am going to a place at the Lord's side, and there I am totally cured."*

For the child and parents, it is important to know that all necessary care will be given and that pain and discomfort will be treated and supervised by the healthcare team from the hospital. Likewise, the relationships with the healthcare team need to gradually unwind when living the last phase of life as normally as possible. Preferably, a few trusted professionals who know the child and family from diagnosis onwards keep regular contact with them by telephone, home visits, and occasional hospital visits. I feel that in the process of ending a life, the child and family must rely on their inner circle. When psychological treatment is requested for a dying child with someone unfamiliar, I think it is wise to be reserved. In my view, there must be overriding arguments to let a dying child invest in a new relationship. The child could best be spared from expending this energy by having the psychological support mediated by familiar members of the healthcare team that tend to the palliative treatment.

How can you live on after your child has died? It is the most difficult, almost impossible task in a parent's life and its difficulty is reflected in the fact that more couples split up after a child dies of leukaemia than when a child is cured. A parent provides a glance behind the scenes, offering insight into this difficult process:

> *"When you have something to celebrate, you're in it together. But when you are down and out, you have to face it alone."*

All's Well that Ends Well?

Children with leukaemia and their families keep looking forward, eager for the end of treatment. When this milestone is reached, the big waiting begins — whether or not the disease will recur. Small numbers of leukaemic cells can cause a relapse of the disease during as well as after cessation of treatment. Because of the likelihood of a relapse, patients are monitored over a prolonged period of time. Long after the cessation of therapy, parents are anxious about the recurrence of the disease.

> *"There is still this anxiety, you know. Every cold, sneezing twice, and you blow up."*

In addition, children can be afraid that the illness might return (Fig. 18). Moreover, parents wonder if the physical side effects will appear in their child.

> *"Something happens all the time. Now they've begun to keep these growth curves, because they've recently found out that these children appear to be behind in growth after all. What will crop up next year? You're always preoccupied about something that might happen, all these problems coming on top of it all. That doesn't stop when treatment is completed."*

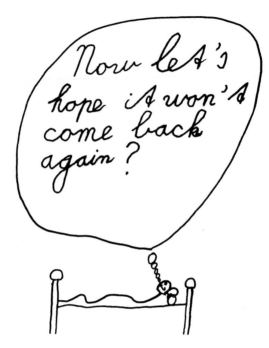

Fig. 18. Wietse's drawing. Children surviving leukaemia may worry whether the illness will return. Even when they have been declared cured, they may doubt whether that is really true. Wietse is 9 years old.

Survival rates have increased with new therapies, which also cause new side effects. For children who respond unfavourably to chemotherapy or for children who relapse, bone marrow transplantation (BMT) is an option. However, the preparation of children for BMT consists of intensive chemotherapy most often combined with total body irradiation that causes unwanted side effects such as infertility. As an 8-year-old girl explained, *"My mother told me that I can't have children anymore. She says, 'you can't have children,' and then my mother tells me that I can just adopt one. Well, I just don't like that, because then you have to adopt children on purpose and it's just so much nicer to have a child of your own."*

Preventive treatment of the central nervous system (CNS) has made a major contribution to the increased survival rates in leukaemia. The first curative therapy included cranial irradiation (see Donald Pinkel's chapter). Short-term follow-up of these children did not reveal serious side effects; however, as the time since cranial irradiation increased, a significant decline in IQ was detected, with younger children being most affected. As an 11 year old survivor of leukaemia pointed out:

My wisdom has gone because of the radiation. That is not why I went to that school in town: a good school for slow learners.

These consequences prompted clinicians to search for other methods with less toxic sequela but with the same or even better survival chances. It was shown that children with forms of CNS preventative treatment other than cranial irradiation did not have more learning problems than children with other forms of cancer who did not receive any form of preventative CNS treatment or their healthy peers.

It is understandable that children and their families have problems with the major late side effects such as a decline in IQ or infertility. However, minor side effects, as compared to the seriousness of the disease, such as dental damage, scaring and problems with hair growth, had more impact than expected. As told by a mother, *"Because she had to take that medicine, it affected her tooth enamel. I didn't like that you know. The child was completely cured but now there is still something permanent."* The reason for this is that the leukaemia experience cannot be tucked away and left behind because these side effects are a constant reminder of the disease for the parent and child.

Upon hearing the potentially fatal diagnosis of leukaemia, the parent's only wish is that their child will live. Now that survival has been accomplished, one would expect them to be relieved, even elated. However, the picture that arises is somewhat different. Instead of happiness, persistence of problems and feelings of loss come to the foreground. First, there are losses in the outlook on life.

> *"You are downright disappointed in life, in the things you believe in."*
>
> *"I really enjoy this world, but that one little thing I had always imagined, a little family that runs smoothly, that should be fine, that should be in harmony, that's been upset. How can I make that clear to you? It's not what it used to be, it will never be like that, it has changed; those days are gone and will never come back."*

In addition, they feel more vulnerable to traumatic events. When confronted with new stresses in life, their psychological balance is more easily disturbed, as is explained by a conversation between parents:

> Mother: *"But then, just like three months ago, when something happens, you find that you unconsciously still have all kind of worries."*
>
> Father: *"That you're vulnerable."*
>
> Mother: *"That you are very vulnerable indeed, when only the slightest thing happens, seemingly, it evokes such clear associations. Then, there you go again."*

Parents experience another loss that concerns the loss of a part of their life. Taking care of a child with leukaemia involves a large amount of time that they could have spent differently if their child had not been ill.

> *"That's a period when you just keep going, you have to, but it certainly cost a few years of our life and we are still making up for those lost years."*

Last but not least, parents can be confronted with losses with respect to their child. As a result of the physical and/or psychological aftermath, parents have to live with the fact that the child is cured of leukaemia, but is not the same child as before the diagnosis:

> *"A number of things in his development have been sped up. We've said from the beginning, 'he'll be getting older sooner; he'll miss part of his youth.' I suppose that's happened. And that's a pity, isn't it, that's bad, that's really a shame."*

A mother of a child with severe neuropsychological deficits: *"We have been given back quite a different child."*

Despite the fact that their child has survived leukaemia, mourning processes in the parents are still induced as a result from losses. These involve various losses addressed above, among which are the psychological impacts that result from the entire process they have undergone. It is unlikely that parents themselves or their social environment recognize these mourning processes or understand why they are not blissful in view of the fact that their child has survived the disease. Although these losses for parents are of a less severe nature compared to the loss they would have experienced if their child died, they nevertheless do affect parents. Thus, with the "choice" between *chance for survival* or *death*, the process involved in completing successful treatment is in fact having chosen the lesser of two evils when one takes into account the challenges parents have met during this drastic, unexpected life event with its long-term effects.

Better or Worse Off by the Experience with Leukaemia?

There is a continuing controversy about the psychological effects after surviving childhood leukaemia. There is a belief that children come out stronger from the illness-experience and even surpass their original capabilities. Moreover, it is often emphasized that the studies on the impact of leukaemia should not only focus on the negative consequences, but also on its positive aspects. It is beyond doubt that children are resilient. It is also true that the adverse experiences inherent in leukaemia can alter the course of the child's development. Due to the illness-experience, children have had to use other "tools" or capabilities to survive psychologically, meaning that some of their abilities are better formed and more honed in comparison with healthy children. Furthermore, survivors may perceive problems differently because they now use a different internal standard to evaluate problems. Daily difficulties and setbacks may be viewed from a different perspective because these are appraised against the experience of having had a life threatening disease. In psychological terms, this "response shift" may explain the lay observations that children with cancer have grown "wise beyond their age."

Parents have also reported positive changes, such as personal growth, appreciation of life, and a more gratifying relationship with their spouse and child. However, the number of positive changes and the few families that experience them requires one to reconsider the status of these gains and examine what meaning they have for the individual. When talking with children and their families, they indicate that the gains from leukaemia and its ensuing treatment *do not compensate* for the hardship and losses caused by the illness. Assigning a positive label to childhood leukaemia may be a way of giving meaning to an extremely stressful life event. It can be regarded as a natural coping response to a universal human need to give meaning to a senseless ordeal. It may be speculated that in emphasizing positive changes, researchers and healthcare professionals may serve their own need to find a meaning for such traumatic experiences. It can be difficult to come to terms with the other side of being cured, especially for paediatric oncologists who are confronted with the late adverse effects of treatment.

In contrast to the belief that children are even better off from having survived leukaemia, it is well established in the literature that the nature and duration of stresses associated with leukaemia or with a chronic physical condition in general, put children at risk for developing psychosocial problems as a late effect. In comparison with healthy children, significantly more serious emotional problems are found in survivors, although this involves a minority. It must be stressed that, in general, the psychological functioning of children who have survived leukaemia is one of psychological normalcy rather than deviance *and*, at the same time, they might still experience feelings and thoughts about having had leukaemia that negatively affect their quality of life. The presence of these long-term psychological consequences underlines the plea to make leukaemia less traumatic for children.

Alleviating Stressors

The challenge is to make childhood leukaemia less distressing by attacking the two major distinctive stressors in leukaemia: the threat of death and the adverse side effects of treatment. All fields involved in treating children with leukaemia, medicine, biology, genetics, and clinical psychology can contribute to this aim by searching for improvements in medical diagnostics, therapy and treatment procedures in order to enhance the prognosis or to diminish the burden of treatment. For instance, a breakthrough in medical research to detect small numbers of leukaemic cells led to substantial reductions of medication intensity for a large subgroup of children with leukaemia, thereby improving the quality of life for these children. Clinical psychology can also help make leukaemia less agonizing for children by dealing with the negative emotions and discomfort related to leukaemia and its treatment, as will be addressed in the last sections of this chapter.

Supporting the parents is helping the child

Parents are the most important source of support and strength for children. If they perceive that their parents can cope with the situation, children will have confidence that the situation is manageable, regardless of how bleak the situation may be. For children, it is important to notice that parents have control over their emotions, otherwise, they will not share with their parents what burdens them. If parents have difficulties in coping with the illness experience, this can block communication between parents and child:

> "*I sometimes talk about it, but then my mother suddenly stops and says: 'perhaps you can do some shopping for me' or something like that.*"

> "*You would like to tell them (parents) what is going on in your head, but then you think: I won't ask them, because they're are going to be so terribly sad and then their whole day is ruined.*"

> "*Well, my mother tells me: 'just don't think about it, I'll tell you later'.*"

Children react to their parents' worries and anxieties; hence, parents may need help in dealing with the situation. They need to help themselves first before they can help their children. In the same way, parents need to know that communication will be hindered if they wish to share *their* worries with their children, which unfortunately, is the advice they receive at times. Therefore, the first step in helping children with leukaemia is helping their parents to care for their own emotions.

There are several ways of empowering parents, for example, by counselling, giving information on how to discuss leukaemia with their children and what they can do to support themselves in dealing with emotions, discomfort, pain and other side effects from medical procedures and therapy. In addition, it is useful to inform parents about parent organizations where parents can find social support from fellow-sufferers. Another issue they need to learn about is how the innate parent-child dynamics involve the instinctive need to help each other. A very important and frequently overlooked issue related to this involves teaching them how to explain to all of their children, their ill child as well as siblings what is helpful to parents and what parents expect and would like them to do. This gives children a sense that they can continue to contribute to family life and that they do not have to feel guilty if they are enjoying themselves by participating in their usual activities. If this is not stated explicitly, the support from children to their parents often goes unnoticed:

> *"Because you know it is also difficult for them (parents) and when they ask 'do you want to continue playing this game?' You just say 'yes', because then they have some diversion as well."*

Helping children to help themselves

Having a life threatening disease is imbued with painful emotions. As explained earlier, children cannot always appropriately express their concerns and emotions because of their developmental level. Besides, they may not want to burden their parents and hence, a neutral person such as a child psychologist can help. In working with children with leukaemia and their siblings, it is useful to start teaching them about feelings in general. I think it is very helpful to explain to them the natural feelings a child can have in a particular situation. It is also helpful to show them that a situation can bring forth different emotions depending on how one thinks about that situation. Often, books in which drawings about feelings in day-to-day situations are depicted could be used to explore their own feelings in general, and subsequently, their feelings related to leukaemia. When children notice that other children can have the same feelings, albeit in different situations, it helps them to recognize their own feelings and that it is normal to have them. When they learn about their own feelings, they may feel less odd and lonely.

I find it beneficial to use books in which situations or feelings are not directly related to the illness-experience. If responding to their actual situation is still too painful, a neutral story provides children a "royal" way out so they can avoid negative feelings or reveal them indirectly. A number of these books that parents and professionals can use are included in the general reference list below (References 6–14). In the same manner, story-telling techniques, also used in play, role-playing, writing and drawing, are very useful to the child psychologist. A whole range of psychotherapeutic techniques are available that focus on expressing emotions and problem solving in order to assist children to come to terms with their emotions. These techniques especially help children find out for themselves how they feel, find out how they can change these feelings, and increase their sense of control. It may be regarded as a kind of antidote to an illness that is characterised by the loss of control and feeling helpless. I find it wonderful to watch children discover what exactly made them feel worse, what helps them to feel better, and to see how proud they are to be better equipped to deal with difficult situations. Their ideas and original solutions are a continuous source of pleasure and inspiration. The technical reference list for a clinical audience contains some books on child psychotherapy, which are suggested as a starting point.

Making treatment less upsetting

The medical procedures used in leukaemia treatment, such as bone marrow aspirations, lumbar and venous punctures, injections, and infusions of chemotherapeutic agents are painful and distressing for the child. The side effects from chemotherapy, such as mouth ulcers, nausea and (anticipatory) vomiting, can also be painful and distressing. There are several methods to control discomfort and pain, including medications and psychological methods. Often, a combination of methods implemented simultaneously achieve the most effect. Several clinical psychological methods that have demonstrated a reduction of pain and discomfort are relaxation, distraction, imagery, hypnosis, and cognitive behavioural techniques.

Nowadays, high dosages of corticosteroids are used in the treatment protocols for leukaemia to obtain better survival rates. However, corticosteroids, in particular dexamethasone, have adverse side effects on mood and behaviour causing sleep disorders, obsessive appetite, irritability, mood swings and unpleasant feelings in the child. These behavioural side effects are of such a severe nature that they are one of the greatest sources of stress during treatment, as a parent explains:

> *"Cancer is the worst part. You're afraid that your child won't survive and dealing with that anxiety is very difficult. Immediately afterwards, come the changes caused by the dexamethasone. You want your child to get better, but it is very difficult to deal with these changes. It just had a great impact on your life. The baldness, the nauseas, being miserable, those you can accept. This change in behaviour is something else. You get another child because of the dexamethasone, but that's the child that goes home with you."*

These medications are administered during a number of consecutive days followed by a period without corticosteroids. The side effects wax and wane according to the therapy schedule and they are tolerated because few medical alternatives are available. The increased survival rates as well as the behavioural side effects are clearly linked to dexamethasone.

I had learned that the appearance and disappearance of behavioural side effects were directly related to the intermittent intake of dexamethasone. This had caused me to conclude that they could not be influenced: that was so, until a 4-year-old girl with leukaemia was referred to me with severe behavioural effects from dexamethasone. She had difficulty falling asleep and often awakened during the night, frequently wanting to eat at that time too. During the day, she was overfatigued, unpleasant, listless, easily irritated and angry. These side effects were present during both the dexamethasone period *and* the corticosteroid-free weeks, albeit to a lesser extent. With this new revelation, I then reasoned that if these side effects were present in the period without dexamethasone, they were being maintained by factors other than the medication. There must be external factors in the child's surroundings, that is, in her immediate environment, which sustain these behavioural problems. If this assumption was to be true, then I could try to influence these factors with clinical psychological methods. The most important people in children's environments are their parents. Accordingly, I described to her parents how behaviour could be shaped and I explained how they could help their child to cope with the side effects of dexamethasone. As a result of further intervention, the sleeping problem reduced sharply. The percentage of nights that the child slept through the night increased from 4 percent before the behavioural therapy treatment to 64 percent after the treatment. In addition, from having registered her sleeping behaviour, the parents also noticed that their child slept more hours. Furthermore, the defiant and irritated behaviour during the day declined, probably as a positive side effect of the improved night time rest. At the follow-up three months after the treatment, it turned out that the positive changes had been maintained.

I was delighted that psychological methods could be effective and started to unravel the underlying mechanism. Learning theory dictates that the environment affects every type of behaviour, independent of its origin. So behavioural side effects, even though they are caused by medications, can be influenced. Although the emotional and behavioural changes in the child are primarily the result of corticosteroids, learning processes determine how these behavioural changes will evolve. Consequently, the child's immediate environment, i.e. the parents, plays an important role in reducing or enhancing behavioural changes caused by dexamethasone. From these premises, we developed a training program for parents on how to cope with the behavioural side effects in their child using classical and operant conditioning principles (see Technical References). The training program considerably reduces the burden of the adverse behavioural effects for the children and their parents. It also improves their quality of life, especially when a child is treated with corticosteroids over an extended period of time.

> "*My life just stood still for two and a half weeks (during the use of corticosteroids). I never had any relaxation in those two weeks. The family is calmer now because of these consultations. Coincidentally, yesterday evening I was reading previous entries in the journal (registration exercise). I thought, 'wow, that was a difficult time for us.' I got a lot out of the training, and I'd recommend it to everyone. In fact, it should be included in the dexamethasone information leaflet.*"

Concluding Remarks

Over the years, I have witnessed that the introduction of more advanced diagnostic and therapeutic methods resulted in more children surviving leukaemia. However, there is a continuous battle between the gains and the sacrifices involved in these new approaches. In search for better survival chances, I think one is obliged to assess the sacrifices involved with these new strategies in the short-term and the long-term and explore how they can be reduced. Clinical psychological methods can contribute to a better quality of life; hence, they must be implemented in order to attain this goal.

Clinical psychological treatment of stressors inherent in the disease and its treatment is still not addressed in the treatment protocols on childhood leukaemia. The exclusion of psychological treatment from standard treatment protocols unfortunately results in the deployment of clinical child psychologists only within the treatment centres that established this as a priority. In addition, a frequently overlooked component is that psychologists have different qualifications, as is the case in medicine. Even though research psychologists have performed psychosocial research in treatment centres in recent decades, clinical child psychologists who are qualified to treat these children and their families are sparse. Most pertinent in this matter is that these professionals have the expertise in how the stressors that are well documented by psychosocial research can be reduced with psychological treatment. Bridging the gap between research findings and clinical practice, along with making sure that psychological treatment becomes an integral part of the medical treatment, regimen, are the challenges for paediatric psychology in the years to come. It is my hope that a closer collaboration among paediatric oncologists, medical scientists, and clinical child psychologists facilitates a growing awareness of the need for psycho-medical treatment regimens to make childhood leukaemia more bearable for the children as well as their families.

Acknowledgement

A special thanks to the children for their drawings.

General References

1. Bluebond-Lagner M, *The Private Worlds of Dying Children*, Princeton University Press, Princeton, 1978.
2. Gordon Th, *Parent Effectiveness Training*, Wijder, New York, 1970.
3. McGrath PJ, Finley GA, Turner CJ, *Making Cancer Less Painful. A Handbook for Parents*, Izaak Walton Killam Children's Hospital and Dalhousie University, Halifax NS, 1992.
4. Sourkes BM, *The Deepening Shade. Psychological Aspects of Life-threatening Illness*, University of Pittsburg Press. Pittsburgh PA, 1982.
5. Van Dongen-Melman JEWM, All is well that ends well!? *Leukemia* **11**: 1197–1200, 1997.
6. Gravett E, *Little Mouse's Big Book of Fears*, Macmillan Publishers, London, 2007.
7. Moses B, Gordon M, *I'm Worried*, Wayland Publishers, Hove, England, 1997.
8. Moses B, Gordon M, *I'm Lonely*, Wayland Publishers, Hove, England, 1997.
9. Moses B, Gordon M, *It's Not Fair*, Wayland Publishers, Hove, England, 1997.

10. Oram H, Ross T, *The Second Princess*, Andersen Press, London, 1994.
11. Parisot F, *Chez Leopold*, Editions du Rouergue, Rodez, 2000.
12. Ross T, *I Don't Want to Go to Hospital*, Andersen Press Ltd, London, 1999.
13. Varley S, *Badger's Parting Gifts*, Andersen Press, London, 1984.
14. Waddell M, Firth B, *Can't You Sleep, Little Bear?* Walker Books, London, 1988.

Technical References

1. Bruce M, A systematic and conceptual review of posttraumatic stress in childhood cancer survivors and their parents, *Clinical Psychology Review*, **26**: 233–256, 2006.
2. Knell SM, *Cognitive-Behavioral Play Therapy*, Jason Aronson, Northvale, New Jersey/London, 1993.
3. Friedman RD, Storytelling and cognitive therapy with children, *Journal of Cognitive Psychotherapy: An International Quarterly*, **8**: 209–217, 1994.
4. Kendall PC, *Child and Adolescent Therapy. Cognitive-Behavioral Procedures*, Guilford Press, New York/London, 1991.
5. Gardner RA, *Therapeutic Communication with Children. The Mutual Story Telling Technique*, Rowman & Littlefield, Lanham, MD, 1986.
6. Van Dongen-Melman JEWM, Sanders-Woudstra JAR, Psychosocial impact of childhood cancer: A review of the literature, *Journal of Child Psychology and Psychiatry*, **27**: 145–180, 1986.
7. Van Dongen-Melman JEWM, *On Surviving Childhood Cancer. Late Psychosocial Consequences for Patients, Parents and Sibling*, Department of Child Psychiatry, Erasmus University, Rotterdam, 1995.
8. Van Dongen-Melman JEWM, Lodders IZ, Plaisier G, *Treating Steroid-induced Behavioral Side Effects in Children: A Parent-training Program. Manual for Professionals. (available as e-book in 2008)*
9. Van Dongen JJM, Seriu T, Panzer-Grümayer ER *et al.*, Prognostic value of minimal residual disease in acute lymphoblastic leukaemia in childhood, *Lancet* **352**: 1731–1738, 1998.

A MOTHER'S JOURNEY

Nicola Horlick

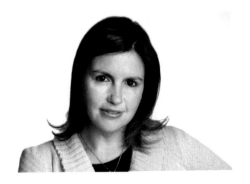

A MOTHER'S JOURNEY

Nicola Horlick

My first child, Georgie, was born in 1986. At the age of 25, I was a relatively young mother by today's standards. I assumed that if the baby was healthy at birth and had all her fingers and toes, then I could look forward to watching her grow up without too much concern. It never occurred to me that I would become the mother of a sick child.

Georgie was a gorgeous baby. She had lovely golden curls and a sunny personality. When she was two years old, she would throw the occasional tantrum, but otherwise, she was a delight. When she was two and a half, we went on holiday with my parents-in-law to Portugal. Then, Georgie developed bronchitis. She was so unwell that we had to call the doctor. Tim, her father and I were very concerned. It was from that moment that Georgie's health began to deteriorate.

Between April and September 1989, we paid many visits to our large general practioner's (GP) clinic. All of the GPs said the same thing. "It's a virus. Don't worry! It'll clear up." Clearly, they thought that I was neurotic and after a while, I began to believe that too. But a mother's instincts are always right when it comes to the health of her child. Despite the constant reassurances by the GPs, I knew that there was something seriously wrong with Georgie and so I took her to see a private doctor in Sloane Street in London. Like the other doctors, he said that there was nothing to worry about and that she would be fine. Eventually, I went back to that doctor and demanded that he do a thorough check up for Georgie. She was then sent for a blood test. That night, she was admitted to the hospital and the next day, she was diagnosed with acute lymphoblastic leukaemia (ALL). She began chemotherapy immediately.

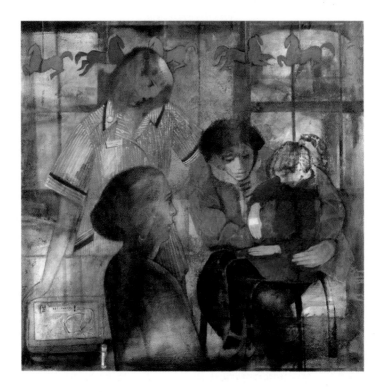

'*Initial Blood Test*' by Susan Macfarlane.

A small child has been referred to the hospital for a blood test and is seen with her mother, nurse and doctor. The blood test requested by the GP is often a precaution to confirm there is little seriously wrong. "*I have chosen the moment just after the blood has been taken and everyone is checking the plaster. The tube of blood is safely on the table behind the doctor.*" In childhood leukaemia some common presenting symptoms are easy bruising, fever, infection, pallor, tiredness, aches and pains especially in the legs and abdomen, and sometimes enlarged glands. Oil on Canvas. 81 × 81 cm. (Courtesy of Euan and Angus Mackay and Dr Geoffrey Farrer-Brown).

Although I knew there was something wrong with Georgie, I was horrified when it became apparent how serious her illness was. I spent a night walking up and down the corridor outside her room, gently weeping. Eventually, a nurse persuaded me to take a sleeping tablet. She told me that I would need lots of energy to deal with the days ahead, and I owed it to Georgie to make sure that I was strong enough for her. Reluctantly, I took the tablet and fell into a deep dreamless sleep. I awoke not really knowing where I was and had to reach into my memory before being confronted again with the horror that was unfolding. I spent another day coming to terms with the shock and then I could feel a force building within me. Georgie needed me to be strong. She needed my support and I had to find out everything that I could about the disease and ensure that she was getting the very best treatment.

Because Georgie was diagnosed by a private doctor, we ended up in a private hospital. I felt uneasy about this but went along with it initially. It was extremely difficult to find out more about acute lymphoblastic leukaemia. There was no internet in those days and after walking around Waterstone's bookshop in Gower Street for hours, I could not find a book that explained the details of the disease or its prognosis. The paediatrician who looked after Georgie when she was born at the very same hospital noticed that Georgie was an in-patient and came into her room to visit us a couple of days after Georgie was diagnosed with ALL. I told him that I was anxious to learn as much as I could about leukaemia and asked if he had anything that I could read to learn about the disease. The next day, he came laden with articles, mostly from the *Lancet*. I was fast beginning to understand the nature of the disease and the treatment that was being used from talking to the nurses and doctors as they administered drugs to Georgie. I read the articles and soon began to decipher them. Eventually, I had sufficient knowledge to be able to work out that we were not necessarily being treated in the right place. One article mentioned the importance of children being treated in specialist centres and that the cure rates were much higher for children who were.

If you are concerned about the treatment that your child is getting in circumstances such as these, what do you do? I called up the Leukaemia Research Fund and talked to its founder, Mr Gordon Piller. He said that I needed to get Georgie into Great Ormond Street Hospital (GOSH) as soon as possible and that he would talk to a professor there. We were lucky. The next day, Professor Judith Chessells saw Georgie and agreed to take her as a patient. I was concerned at first as she said that she would have to get hold of Georgie's file and see if she had had appropriate treatment. We spent a few days anxiously waiting for Judith to pronounce on this. Eventually, she said that the treatment had been appropriate, although a third block of chemotherapy, which had originally been planned, had not been administered. She felt that this would have been better but assured us that it was not the end of the world.

Thereafter, I felt much happier. Georgie was clearly in the hands of some of the most competent paediatric doctors in the world. She had two years of maintenance treatment and then came off all medication. She was then five and was lively and intelligent. Once she stopped chemotherapy, her hair started growing. She looked like any other five year old.

Between the ages of five and eight, Georgie was totally well and we were approaching the time when the doctors would declare her cured. In April 1995, we went skiing in France and Georgie felt very unwell. As the days went by, she became listless. Worried that she may be sick, I called the doctor. I told him about her medical history. The doctor said that we should go straight to GOSH on our return. I was so anxious that I could not eat or sleep. When I got to GOSH, there were more hours of waiting whilst the doctors analysed the blood sample. Finally, the results came through to the consultant, Dr Alison Leiper, who was familiar with Georgie's case. She said that it all looked fine and that it must be a bug. Later that day, she called to say that they had repeated the analysis of the blood sample again. This time, they concluded that Georgie had suffered a relapse.

Girls who have acute lymphoblastic leukaemia have a better prognosis than boys diagnosed with the disease. The longer the child lives without a relapse, the more likely that she is cured. Georgie had been in remission for five and a half years. How could it be that she had relapsed? Tim and I went through the same feelings that we had when she was first diagnosed. Why her? Why us? At this point, I was an "expert" in leukaemia and I knew my way round the system. However, nothing that I had experienced with Georgie up to that point had prepared me for what was to come.

Shortly after Georgie started on the relapse protocol, she became very unwell. We were living in Hampshire and so she was admitted to the hospital in Winchester. Tim had to go back to work and we asked if we could take her to the Chelsea and Westminster Hospital in London. The doctors agreed that this would be okay. We drove to the Chelsea and Westminster and over the following few days, Georgie's condition deteriorated further. An angry red patch had developed on her right buttock and then it spread to her left buttock. The doctors at that hospital did not seem particularly concerned about her condition but I was becoming increasingly hysterical. Eventually, I called Dr Alison Leiper who arranged for Georgie to be taken to GOSH in an ambulance at once.

Georgie was near to death by the time she arrived at GOSH. She had necrotising faciitis, a deadly flesh eating disease. A surgeon came into her room and said that she would be taken to the operating theatre immediately and that they would have to cut away the infected flesh. It was highly likely that she would have a cardiac arrest on the operating table. However, if she survived, she would be admitted to intensive care immediately. Clinging to each other for comfort, Tim and I stayed in her room on the main ward whilst the operation took place. We were somewhat amazed when Georgie was brought back to her room alive. She had pulled through and the doctor decided that it was unnecessary for her to go to intensive care.

The surgeon had cut away two thirds of Georgie's right buttock and one third of her left buttock and she had a colostomy. She was placed on an airbed and was given huge doses of morphine. The wound could not be grafted for a week and so the dressing was stitched to her. Everyday, for seven days, she was brought to the operating theatre. Under general anaesthetic, the wound was cleaned and the dressing replaced. Through the haze of morphine, Georgie, then eight years old, said to me: "Mummy, how can there be a God if he makes a little child like me suffer like this." I had no response to give her.

It is amazing how resilient children are. After weeks of lying on an airbed to the point where her legs had totally wasted, Georgie started to walk and eat again. She insisted on going back to school and the headmistress and staff had to carry her up and down the stairs for the first few days. But after a week, she was running around again. Georgie felt conscious having no hair at the age of eight, so she decided to try a wig. The wig shop did not have a strawberry blonde wig, but they very kindly gave her a dark wig and another blonde one. She insisted on wearing the blonde wig when she returned to school and was very upset when no one recognised her. The next day, the wigs went into the dressing up box.

There were ups and downs with Georgie's treatment as the relapse protocol progressed, but she got through it and then had another two years of maintenance treatment. She came off the drugs in April 1997 and was very well for the next seven months before relapsing again. At this point, we knew that it was a very serious situation. It was bad enough relapsing once. A second relapse would be very difficult to deal with. A bone marrow transplant would be the only option.

A search of the bone marrow donor register showed that there were two good matches for Georgie from unrelated donors. Despite the fact that we had four other children, none of them were a match. In the end, this was seen as a good thing as the doctors felt that a sibling donor would not have provided enough fight against what was clearly a very virulent form of the disease. We were told that male donors were preferred to female donors who had had children and we had one of each, so it was the male donor who was chosen. All we knew was that he was in his forties and lived in the Bristol area. We were not allowed to know his identity.

Having established that there was a donor, the doctors at GOSH had to get Georgie into remission again. I assumed that this would happen with relative ease but I was wrong. The first lot of treatment did not work and so she had to have a block of very heavy duty drugs which eventually did the trick. I was taken aside by one of the consultants who told me that the fact that it had been so difficult to get Georgie into remission was a poor prognostic indicator and that we should bear this in mind. Things did not look particularly good but we had no choice but to proceed with the bone marrow transplant and hope that it would work. However, the intensity of the treatment was beginning to take its toll on Georgie. She was never fat but she was always well covered. She lost about 10 Kgs in weight during this period and was beginning to look very frail. I was very concerned about whether she would be strong enough to deal with the transplant.

Georgie was applying to new schools in the midst of all this. I spoke to her headmistress and asked for her opinion about whether Georgie should wait for a year to take the entrance exams for the four schools she was applying to. The headmistress felt that Georgie should go ahead and take the exams. I then spoke to the high mistress of St. Paul's Girls' School, Georgie's first choice and she agreed. Finally, I asked Georgie herself what she felt and she was appalled by the suggestion that she should defer her applications. She insisted on taking the exams then. Eventually, Georgie sat for three of her entrance papers in her room in GOSH. The final exam was for St. Paul's. At the end of January, on a freezing cold day, Georgie got out of bed, got dressed and I drove her to St. Paul's to take the exam. She felt that the exam was so important that she had to go in person and not take the exam in her room in GOSH. Having left my extremely frail and sick child at St. Paul's, I drove away feeling very apprehensive. I dropped her at 9 a.m. and had to collect her at 3 p.m. I was very worried. Thankfully, she came bouncing down the main steps of the school with a huge smile on her face and told me that it was much easier than she thought it would be. Indeed, Georgie got her place at St. Paul's. All of us were filled with admiration for her determination and courage.

The ward that Georgie was admitted to was filled with complicated cases. It felt like death row. Their parents were demoralised and depressed and it was very difficult to keep our spirits up in such circumstances. In some ways, it was a relief when we were transferred to the bone marrow ward for the transplant. Georgie and I were to be incarcerated in a room alone for ten weeks. I had to cut my hair off, jettison all jewellery other than my wedding band, and try to leave the room as little as possible. I managed to persuade the sister on the ward to allow me to have my computer in the room so that we would have a link with the outside world. In those days, this was an unusual request and there were some objections to my plan, but eventually, it was agreed that we could have the computer.

Georgie began her treatment with total body irradiation. This was a harrowing experience for both of us. Georgie felt very sick despite the anti-nausea drug that she was on. I was concerned about the side effects of the treatment, knowing for sure that she would be infertile as a result and that there would be a risk of her developing other cancers. One major side effect of total body irradiation is a very sore mouth and gut. As a result, Georgie was put on total parenteral nutrition (TPN) and given iced lollies to ease the pain in her mouth. She was on heavy doses of morphine. Georgie never reacted well to morphine. It made her aggressive and she started kicking and hitting me and the nurses. It was so horrible that she had to be switched to pethadine. Pethadine worked but made her extremely drowsy. We were living through a nightmare and I was beginning to wonder how we would survive when things took a turn for the worse.

By this stage, Georgie had had the necessary transplant drugs and the infusion of the donor's marrow. She then developed a very rare condition called haemorrhagic cystitis. Georgie started peeing out

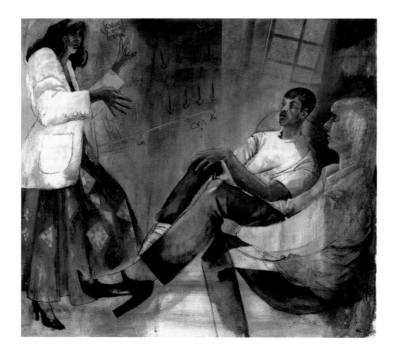

'*First Interview in the Bone Marrow Transplant Unit*' by Susan Macfarlane.
The Bone Marrow Transplant Physician meeting with the parents of a young child and explaining that the suggested treatment for the child's leukaemia is now a bone marrow transplant. All stages of this treatment, including side effects and long term follow up are carefully explained. *"The young couple try to grasp all they are being told. So much to remember and so hard to believe that all this must really happen to their own beloved child."* Oil on Canvas. 76 × 86 cm. (Courtesy of Euan and Angus Mackay and Dr Geoffrey Farrer-Brown).

blood clots which were the size of kidney bowls. Neither Tim nor I had seen anything like that and found it extremely distressing. Georgie's haemoglobin plummeted and she had to have constant blood transfusions. I was at my wits end as none of the doctors seemed to have any suggestions as to how to deal with this condition. I talked to one of the senior nurses and she was very concerned that the condition might kill Georgie. I got hold of the senior registrar on the ward and begged her to try and find a solution. She called Bristol, which is the biggest and most long standing transplant centre in the UK. The doctors there suggested giving Georgie low-dose oral oestrogen. A nurse came in with a pair of surgical stockings — there was a concern about thrombosis as a side effect — and then the course of treatment began. On the seventh day, Georgie got up and peed in the bedpan and there were no blood clots. I ran out of the room and the nurses and I were jumping for joy.

Eventually, Georgie was discharged from the bone marrow unit and we went home. However, her body had taken such a beating from the treatment that she started having renal problems. We were only at home for two days before being readmitted again. Apart from the occasional afternoons at school or at home, Georgie remained in the hospital for the following six months. She had developed bowel difficulties as well as renal problems and had constant diarrhoea. She was denied food and had to live on TPN. Georgie was getting increasingly fed up. This went on remorselessly.

Georgie had relapsed on 5th December 1997 and it was now the middle of November 1998. She spent the previous few weeks making bracelets, necklaces, Christmas cards and other items to sell at her school's Christmas fair. St. Paul's had agreed that she could have her own stall at the fair and that Georgie could give the proceeds to the playroom on her ward in GOSH. On the day of the Christmas fair, I got Georgie up and dressed her and the nurses detached her drip. Tim and I loaded all the things that Georgie had made into the car and drove her to the school. We decorated the stall and got everything ready and a steady stream of people came to buy Georgie's creations. She sold out and raised £350 for the playroom. She was very pleased with herself and Tim and I were extremely proud of her achievement.

The next day, Georgie and I had an extremely sad conversation. She told me that she wanted to go to sleep and never wake up. "How can you say that after all that we have been through, darling?" I asked. She said that she had a poor quality of life. She could not bear the constant diarrhoea and the fact that she could not eat real food. She felt it would be better if she was allowed to go. I sobbed that night as I lay in my bed in her hospital room.

A week later, I came into Georgie's room and noticed a deterioration in her breathing. Tim had been with her during the day and I had been looking after the other children. As the evening went on, her breathing got worse, and she needed oxygen. An X-ray of her lung was taken and I asked if it was aspergillus. Aspergillosis is a fungal infection that all transplant patients, their parents and doctors fear most. Nothing can be done if a patient succumbs to it. It is fatal. The junior doctor said that she could not tell anything from the X-ray and that a consultant would talk to us the next morning.

After a very uncomfortable night, Georgie was taken to the operating theatre the following afternoon. I always felt apprehensive when Georgie had a general anaesthetic, but I knew this time that Georgie might not come out of theatre alive and that, if she did, she would be in the intensive care unit. She survived and we were reunited in the intensive care unit. It was horrifying to see my beloved Georgie on a life support machine, unable to breathe for herself. She had contracted aspergillus and an experimental drug from Belgium would be administered to her. In the meantime, the doctors decided that they would leave her sedated and on the life support machine overnight. Then would try taking her off the life support machine the next day to see if she could breathe for herself.

As I tried to rest in Georgie's room, I could not sleep. I ended up wandering around the hospital corridors trying to comprehend what was happening. I was trying to be honest with myself and had to accept the fact that the end of our long journey was approaching. I went to Georgie's intensive care cubicle and laid my head next to hers, stroking her soft white hand. Tears rolled down my face and the nurse urged me to go back to the ward. I stayed there for two hours, well into the early hours of the morning, crying and crying. Eventually I walked back and spent the rest of the night in an uneasy and tortured sleep.

The next day was the worst of my life and that of Georgie's too. She was taken off the life support machine and was gasping for air. The doctors tried everything, but it was clear that she was unable to breathe on her own. "Help me, Mummy, help me", she said. It was heartbreaking. I tried to distract her from her distress by promising that we would go to New York, ride in yellow cabs and go to the top of the Empire State Building. However, that did not soothe Georgie and she became more and more desperate. Eventually, we had to accept the fact that she needed to go back on the life support machine.

It was clear now that Georgie was going to die. The doctors at GOSH were fantastic and did not make us turn off the life support machine immediately. They allowed us to leave it on for a few more days in order to get used to the idea that Georgie had come to the end of the road. During the following two and a half days, about 60 members of the staff from GOSH filed through her room to say goodbye. Nurses, doctors, psychologists, play specialists, cleaners, people who worked in the shop — they all wanted to say goodbye to the girl they had known for nine years. The girl who had fought so bravely and always had a smile for them even if things were really bad. Professor Judith Chessells came to say goodbye, kissed Georgie and then made the sign of a cross on her forehead. As I recount this, tears are rolling down my face as they were then. We were living out a tragedy. Our beautiful, clever and talented daughter was dying.

We agreed with the doctors that the machine would be turned off at lunchtime on 27th November 1998. I arranged for our local vicar to come and say prayers for Georgie. There were fourteen people in the room including Tim, me, various of our siblings, my mother, my grandmother, most of Georgie's godparents, a couple of cousins and the mother of Georgie's best friend. Only one of our other children wanted to be there — Serena who was then eight years old. After the vicar had finished, I lay across Georgie and held her with Tim and Serena holding onto me. Everyone held hands and wept as the doctor turned off the machine. Georgie had a strong heart and it seemed to take forever for her to die. After some minutes, she was pronounced dead. The long battle had ended and Georgie was free.

When the tubes were removed, I was astonished to see that she had a huge smile on her face. She had got what she wanted and was finally at peace.

Coming to terms with the loss of a child, especially after such a long battle for life, is very difficult. My first concern was for my other four children. Great Ormond Street Hospital provided wonderful support and three of the children (then aged ten, eight and five years old) saw the psychologist who had been responsible for Georgie during her bone marrow transplant and who gave them counselling. The fourth child was only two years old and so it was not deemed necessary for her to have this sort of help. There is no question that all of our children who were alive at the time of Georgie's death have suffered as a result. There is one positive in this in that it has made them very charitable people and I am proud that they are eager to help others who they perceive to be less fortunate than themselves. It is probably too early to guage what the long-term effects will be on them, but I expect that they will be profound.

Sadly, Tim and I split up five years after Georgie died. It is difficult to know whether this was directly attributable to the loss of Georgie, but the statistics definitely suggest that it is very difficult for marriages to survive after a child dies. The divorce placed a huge emotional burden on my family and it was a very tough period for all of us.

Despite the horrors that we suffered as a result of Georgie's illness and death, I feel extremely privileged to have been her mother. Georgie was a wonderful person and I would much rather have had her for twelve years and lost her than not having her at all. I learnt so much from Georgie. She was truly the most remarkable and brave person that I have ever met. Everyone who knew her will remember her and I know that they too learnt a great deal from her. Children who fight illness over a long period have a special quality and wisdom that affects those who come into contact with them.

It is important to try and learn from this type of experience and to look beyond the immediate loss. Georgie was only meant to live for

12 years. She was here for a reason and she made her mark on those around her and taught them a great deal. I know that Georgie would not want me to be an emotional wreck who cannot function. I have to keep going for the other children, but most importantly, I keep going for her.

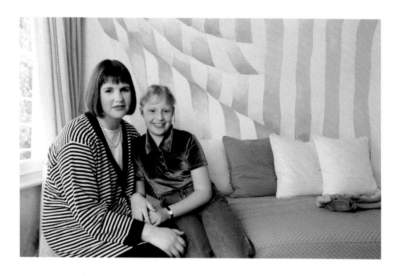

Fig. 19.   Photo of Nicola Horlick with Georgie

A FAMILY'S JOURNEY:
THE CHILD, THE MOTHER

Janine Fernandes, Delena Fernandes

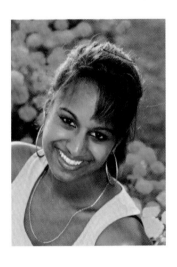
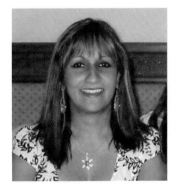

A FAMILY'S JOURNEY: THE CHILD

Janine Fernandes

What does every four year old child enjoy doing? Learning to write, playing in the park with my friends, and going to school; everyday things. I was a typical four year old child, living in Bexley, Kent (the UK) with a mother, father and younger sister. I loved playing with dolls, watching "Sesame Street" on television, and generally being cheerful and giggly. I led a perfectly normal life. However, as a four year old girl suddenly diagnosed with leukaemia, your whole life changes. At the time when I was diagnosed, I changed from being a fun loving youngster to somebody with long bouts of being sad and feeling unwell. This was probably due to the countless number of blood transfusions, blood tests, infections, lumbar punctures, and countless injections. No wonder I was no longer that bubbly child. However, I suppose I should be grateful for the fact that I was not, at that time, in any physical pain.

Recognition and Realisation

I guess my journey really began on the day my Mum had taken my baby sister, Kirsten, to be weighed for the usual routine check up. Only it turned out that it was me, not my sister that needed close examination. My recollection of that day was quite vivid. "She doesn't look too well, Mrs Fernandes" the health visitor murmured. She advised my Mum to see the doctor immediately for a more thorough examination. However, I was oblivious to the extent of the problem at that stage.

I can recall my Mum being very sad and dismal when we left the clinic. I tried to talk to her but I could tell that she was somewhat preoccupied. When we arrived home, I remember Mum speaking with my Dad in a sad and despondent voice. I think those were one of my most poignant moments when I felt that something was not quite right. After that, everything seemed to happen at a very fast pace. I was marched to the doctor's surgery that same evening. I sat with my Mum in the doctor's consulting room, and the only thing I can recall is my Mum asking the doctor "Is there something seriously wrong with her?" The doctor's only response to her was that we needed to take some blood tests so that they could make a proper diagnosis. My poor Mum was resigned to this response.

I remember feeling a sense of unease that night. I am sure my parents were being protective over me. They kept asking me "are you sure you are feeling alright" or "is there anything we can get you?" I kept reassuring them that I was fine but I am sure they did not believe me. I do not remember too much about that particular night but I am pretty sure it must have seemed like a lifetime for my parents until the next morning.

The dreaded morning finally arrived. We drove to Queen Mary's Hospital, Sidcup in silence. None of us knew what to expect. I felt a little scared and anxious at this point. After all, I did not know what was going to happen to me. I think, for me at that stage, it was a sense of not knowing. *What is going to happen to me? Will I be alright?* Questions like these flooded into my head. Questions. Just so many questions. As for my parents, who knows what they were thinking?

Obviously, being a 4 year old, you are unaware of what signs and symptoms led to my diagnosis. However, I do remember feeling a little bit weak, and not having enough energy to do things I had previously done before. I also recall feeling so cold all the time. I remember being at my Godfather's house for a family party. All the children had been playing outside in the sunshine, and I quite candidly said to my Mum "I am feeling really cold". So I came inside the house and I was still very cold so my Godfather put on the central heating for me. However, I just could not warm up. Then there was the time I was at a friend's birthday party and I had a terrible nose bleed. I can recall the parent mentioning this to my Mum when she came to collect me.

We arrived at the hospital. At this stage, none of us knew what it was we would have to face walking through those hospital doors. The corridors seemed like an endless road that led on to nowhere. I felt as if my life was unfolding right before my very eyes; daunting, forbidding and chilling. These are only a few adjectives that even begin to describe what I felt at that precise moment. For my parents, who obviously had experienced much more of life than myself, these emotions must have been intensified about a thousand times. Suddenly, I stopped and pointed out, "Daddy, what's the name of that pretty bird on that branch over there?" Looking back on this moment, it seemed like the least helpful thing to say to either of my parents. My Dad stared into space, preoccupied with some other matter. He looked intently at the bird for a moment and then turned to me. "I'm sorry darling, but I don't know," he whispered, shaking his head solemnly.

All I remember about that day was sitting between my parents and just staring at the pink form clutched tightly in my Mum's hand. The word "**URGENT**" kept jumping out at me from all angles. The rest of the words on the form squirmed on the page like slimy black snakes. The next minute, I was sitting on my Mum's lap in the pathology lab. I can recall my parents trying to calm me down as I sobbed bitterly. I had to have a blood test but I was absolutely terrified of needles. Even to this day, many years on, I have vivid memories of my first blood test. It was a painful procedure for me then as it is still to this day. The waiting, the pain, but then that small plaster after the blood test with Minnie Mouse's face imprinted on it; it made me feel better, or for a while anyway.

I can remember the pained look on both my parents' faces. Anguish seemed to outline their faces. On the way back home, my Dad pulled up outside Woolworth's store. "Janine, as you have been such a brave girl, go and choose any video you want, okay?" he smiled at me. Brave girl? Talk about laying it on thickly! Just a few moments ago, I had been crying my heart out non-stop! Anyhow, I was thrilled. So, jumping out the car, with my tear stained face, I grabbed my Mum's hand, and waltzed into the shop. Typically, I ran over to the children's home video section. There are so many choices! I felt like the luckiest girl alive. "Mummy, look! Aristocats! Yippee!" I yelled, feeling exhilarated. I absolutely loved Disney films, alongside Sesame Street. We paid for the video and made our way back to the car.

As soon as we arrived home, I slid my new video cassette into the recorder and began to watch it. I still had no clue what was going on. As a very young child, I can barely remember how I felt at the time. Perhaps the excitement of watching my favourite film was suppressing my true feelings of anxiety, or maybe I was just too young to understand. At this point, I was surrounded by most of my family. I can recall my grandparents being quieter than their usual lively selves. However, in my presence, they always made an effort to put on a brave smile. Who knows if I was easily fooled or not?

Later that evening, there was a loud knock on the door. For some strange reason, I can remember my heart pounding at a very fast pace. In not so many words, extremely fast. That knock. That dreaded knock. My Mum opened the door gingerly, her hands trembling. "Hello, Mrs Fernandes. May I come in? I have Janine's blood test results from this morning." "What is it Dr Banerjee?" my Mum inquired, looking both tensely and nervously at the doctor. "It's not good news, I'm afraid. The blood test showed abnormal blood cells which suggest it is leukaemia," Dr Banerjee informed my Mum in a shaky voice. There was an awful moment of silence. The doctor advised my Mum to take me to Queen Mary's Hospital the very next day to see a consultant. He left just as my Dad had come down the stairs from having a shower. He noticed my Mum had been crying.

"What's wrong, Delena?" he asked urgently, "What's happened?" The next few moments must have been incredibly difficult for my parents. A few seconds later, my Dad had tears rolling down his face. "Are you sure it was a blood disorder? Why Janine? Why our little Janine?" he kept repeating these words over and over again.

Meanwhile, I was still glued to the latest addition to my video collection. I was surrounded by most of my cousins; all of us perched on the sofa. I had no inkling of what Dr Banerjee had just told my parents. A simple answer to a life changing question? No. I look back now and wonder how I would have felt if I was that much older and knew about leukaemia. My parents did not really speak to me about the day's events. I suppose they did not want to upset me, and moreover, they were trying to come to terms with what had happened themselves. The question was even if my parents had tried to explain the situation to me, would I have had any grasp of the situation and would I have understood the seriousness of it all?

The next day, I found myself outside the hospital again. I did wonder if this was going to become a regular occurrence. I remember a short man in a white coat approaching my Mum and Dad. It seemed like a lifetime waiting for him to come and fetch us. My Mum and Dad looked decidedly uncomfortable. It is only now that I can appreciate what thoughts and emotions they must have been going through. Imagine being told that your four year old daughter has been diagnosed with leukaemia. I have vague memories of that moment when Dr Saad Rassam took us into his consulting room. I do remember being perched on my Mum's knee, though. It seemed to me like we were in there for ages. I suppose my Mum and Dad had to ask Dr Rassam all the obvious if difficult questions. I was oblivious to what was happening around me at that time but I felt it was something to be worried and anxious about. I do recall Dr Rassam explaining to my parents in great detail what leukaemia was, the chances of cure or my prognosis, and the course of treatment that needed to be followed. I do not think my parents could take in all the information. They looked somewhat bewildered and who could blame them.

Next, Dr Rassam examined me. He seemed friendly and he was very gentle with me. He asked me how I was feeling and I said to him not very well. After his thorough examination, he let me sit back on my Dad's lap. My parents watched as Dr Rassam made some notes in a large, pink folder for a few moments. Then, there was a dreadful silence. My Dad was the first to speak. "Can she be cured? Or is she going to…" My Dad's voice trailed off to a whisper. The words would just not come out. Dr. Rassam shook his head. "No, Mr. Fernandes. I can assure you that we will give Janine the best treatment possible, in order for her to fight this leukaemia." Both at the time and during my treatment, I never grasped the fact, or even suspected, that leukaemia could be lethal.

Diagnosis

So, here I was in a consulting room being told I had this horrible disease and at the same time feeling unwell and weak. I had not even completed preschool. Now, I was in hospital not knowing if I would even make it to my first day at primary school. At that time I certainly did not realise how ill I actually was. Dr Rassam contacted Lamorbey Ward, the children's ward at the hospital and explained the situation to them. I was to be admitted after our consultation with Dr Rassam. As soon as I entered the ward, I was greeted by two Irish nurses, Jane and Carol. They were the most loving and caring nurses I have ever met. Both of them had a vast amount of experience of working with children with cancer when they worked in Ireland. In addition to caring for me, they supported my parents throughout my battle against leukaemia. One could say they educated my Mum and Dad on leukaemia. As I settled into my room, I can remember that my parents were handed a stack of leaflets and various other pamphlets by Jane and Carol. To this day, my parents are eternally grateful to them because through the bewilderment, anxiety and stress of discovering about my diagnosis, both Jane and Carol advised, supported and comforted them.

Nurse Jane — well what can I say about her? She was my nurse as well as my adult friend. I am sure Jane could read my mind because she instinctively knew that I was scared and unsure of what was going to happen to me next. So to help me understand my condition and what would happen to me next, she produced a small doll and placed it in front of me. Wow, I thought to myself, more toys! Jane sat on the edge of my bed and smiled at me. Taking the doll as a person, she explained to me, in simple terms, what would happen to me next. She explained to me that I was not very well at the moment but after various injections and some medicine I would be feeling like a new person. Next, she placed a thermometer in the doll's mouth and emphasized to me that she and other nurses would need to keep taking my temperature in order to work out how unwell I was. By this stage, and due to the warm, caring attitude of my two wonderful nurses, Jane and Carol, I felt quite at ease with what treatment had to follow.

Do you remember what I said to you about that first injection not being my last? Well, I could not have been more right. No sooner had I settled down in my hospital bed, I was whisked off to another hospital room with yet more nurses and doctors. Not two more injections. Not three. Not even four, but five more injections were given to me. It felt as if ten thousand knives were stabbing me all over my body at once. I cried in the exact same way that I cried during my first blood test. My Mum, who had sat with me through these many injections, must have felt as if her insides were being ripped out of her. I kept thinking to myself how many more of these injections do I have to go through. I can recall trying to stare at the Eeyore Donkey poster on the opposite wall, just as the nurse had told me. But, I ask you honestly, how is any young child confronted with the prospect of having needle after needle inserted into their bodies supposed to be cool, calm and collected?

That same night, it was my Dad who stayed with me in hospital. My Mum had hurried back home to collect some of my favourite belongings such as my Charlotte dolly and my Mickey Mouse cuddly toy. All the things a regular four year old would want with them at all times. My parents felt at least these familiar things would bring me some comfort in an unfamiliar environment.

Treatment

I survived that first day but was very much unaware of what was to follow. At that moment in time I had no idea about the nightmare I would have to endure. The word "nightmare" does not even begin to describe how I felt those first few days. Scared, anxious and feeling weak and vulnerable, that's how I would describe myself.

The second day was positively worse than the first. I had to have my first lumbar puncture. To any child, a lumbar puncture would have been something possibly associated with a car tyre. Well, I can tell you, in medical terms, a lumbar puncture is a diagnostic procedure that is performed in order to collect a sample of cerebrospinal fluid from the spine. I know that my Mum could not face being in the room with me because it was just too painful for her to sit and watch. The lumbar puncture was crucial to my treatment because it would ascertain how far the leukaemia had spread and what course of treatment would be administered to me. Once the results of the lumbar puncture came through a few days later, it indicated that the leukaemia had not spread to my spinal cord which meant I had a very positive prognosis. Following this, Dr Rassam informed my parents of the treatment which would follow.

I had shared care treatment which meant I had the initial chemotherapy treatment at Queen Mary's Hospital. I've since been told that this consisted of an intravenous chemotherapy drug called vincristine, and then another one called asparaginase, which was injected into my right leg. I can recall it was a very painful injection, the needle being inserted into my thigh. By that point, I had lost so much weight that I felt the pain even more so. Besides this, I had to have blood tests, blood transfusions, platelet transfusions, and oral treatment for thrush. However, on the 1st June 1995, I began my main chemotherapy treatment at Great Ormond Street Hospital (GOSH) in London. What this usually meant for me was that I had my intensive blocks of chemotherapy treatment for a period of six days. This consisted of very strong and powerful drugs including prednisolone and cotrimoxazole. I would then come home to recover from the treatment. However, this would not last for long as I would become very ill with one infection or another as my immune system was so low and I would end up going back to Queen Mary's in Sidcup five days later. At this particular point, my body could not withstand any sort of infection. I would become weak, pale, exhausted and almost lifeless at times.

I know I had many highs and lows during my hospital stays. I remember feeling so weak that I could barely lift my head off the pillow. I had high temperatures, bouts of vomiting, diarrhoea and many other side effects from the cocktail of drugs. However, the one good thing was that I know that I was thoroughly spoilt as a result of all of this suffering. There was nothing more a child could want for. When I was feeling well and my blood counts were good, I was allowed to receive visitors. You have never seen so many presents in all your life. I received teddy bears, books, videos, dolls, balloons, sweets, chocolates, colouring books and pencils, and many games to keep me occupied during my stay in hospital. I remember thinking to myself at one point that it was not such a bad thing being ill. However, I did realise at that point there was a downside to being ill as well.

During the course of my two year treatment, I experienced many side effects. However, the most vivid of those memories are the times when I was put under general anaesthetic in order for me to undergo a lumbar puncture. These lumbar punctures were a crucial part of my treatment. I received one after every block of chemotherapy treatment to ensure that the leukaemia was not spreading. This procedure was carried out in order for the doctors to test whether there were any leukaemic cells in my spinal cord, and at the same time the doctors would administer a drug called methotrexate to me while I was under general anaesthetic. I can recall the nurses' and my parents' faces fading right before my very eyes within a matter of seconds. Before I knew it, I was out for the count. I can remember so vividly to this day the abnormal dreams I experienced whilst this procedure was being carried out on me. They are vague memories now but they appeared to be colourful animations floating in my mind. I also saw familiar faces, such as my parents; they looked to me as if they were constructed out of Lego pieces which kept wading in and out of my dream. At the time, my parents did explain to me as best as they could, in a child-like language, that I had to have these lumbar punctures in order for the doctors to make sure that the cancer cells were leaving my body once and for all. Since it was explained to me by my parents in this manner, I felt I could handle it and also the fact that it was something that had to be done to make me better again.

Besides my many stays in hospital, I had to attend the outpatients department at the local hospital and the long term follow-up clinic at GOSH frequently. These visits are a regular reminder to me that I should still not take life for granted. If it is not a blood test, it is a heart echo, if it is not a heart echo, then it is being weighed in and if it is not a weigh in, then it is a check up with one of the consultants. It is just an endless stream of tests, treatments, scans and more consultations with the doctors. I know it had to be done but it does not make it any easier to bear. So one could say that I spent the majority of the early part of my life in a hospital. I have to say that the best part of my hospital stays were the many friends I made at the hospital, such as the receptionists in the pathology laboratory, the nurses and the doctors. They have seen me grow up from a weak and poorly 4 year old to an independent and healthy 17 year old. Some of them say to me that they cannot believe the years have gone by so quickly. I tell them I am glad it has gone quickly, without wishing my life away.

On the odd occasions I was able to stay at home, I would still have the McMillan nurses coming in to take blood from me to be tested at the local hospital to ensure that my blood counts were doing ok. However, I have to say I am eternally grateful to these nurses because it enabled me to have some sort of family life at home. It saved the journey yet again to the hospital for my parents, who by now must have been very tired and weary, though they never showed it. They always had a smile on their faces and this carried me through the really hard times.

While in hospital receiving treatment, I can remember being inundated with cards and paintings from the children in my reception class. For a few moments, the swirling splotches of yellow and green paint would almost dissolve the pain of having a permanent drip attached to my arm. Alongside emla cream, the drip became another good friend of mine. Whenever I felt bored, I would stand on the base of the machine and my Dad would wheel me up and down that long hospital corridor. At the time, I thought it was terrific and the most fun thing I had ever done. My Dad, I'm sure, was thinking otherwise.

Hair Loss and Havoc

I think the worst part of my whole treatment was the fact that I had to lose my long dark wavy hair. For any four year old and especially for a girl, their hair is their pride and joy. When that was taken away from me, I felt as if I was being stripped of my femininity. To me, that time, it was only boys who had their hair shaved. I looked like a boy! I felt abnormal. Would people stare at me and wonder if I was a boy? Would people wonder what was wrong with me? Up to the point before my hair loss, no one would have guessed that I was ill. Now, everyone would know.

As a child, I felt a deep sadness and resentment of the fact that this disease not only took away my life from me but it also took away my looks as well. I felt as if I was no longer me. I felt some sort of turmoil going on inside me and it made me terrified to even think of the future. When I lost my hair, everything changed. *I* changed both physically and emotionally.

After several blocks of chemotherapy at GOSH, my hair started falling out bit by bit. I even remember the time I was playing with my baby sister, Kirsten, on the floor and something had fallen underneath the kitchen cabinets. So, I put my head down to see if I could fetch it for her, when all of a sudden, she just placed her hand on a bit of my long hair; a clump had just come off. I remember my Mum shouting at her, although it was not her fault at all. Although my Mum felt sorry for me and Kirsten but there was no way we could put it back on my head. So yet again, I had lost some more hair. I would sleep with a white sheet on my bed and in the mornings when I woke up, the whole sheet would be covered in hair. One day, it was so bad that my Mum and Dad sat down with me and explained that I was going to lose all my hair anyway. They explained that, at that time, it looked odd for me to have bits of hair here and there and none in some other spots. They said it would be better if they were to shave it all off and then it could grow nice and thick again. I agreed, hesitantly. So there we were in the middle of the garden. My Dad with a hair razor with one hand ready to go for the kill. Slowly but slowly, I watched tuft of hair by tuft of hair falling to the ground around me. I felt a sick feeling inside me. This was really it. I was going to be bald. I was worried that my hair would never grow back. I saw the sadness in my Mum's eyes. I knew that she wanted to cry but she would not do it in front of me. She said I looked the sweetest, cutie pie ever. That did make me feel very proud, for a moment anyway.

I no longer felt comfortable going out with my parents in public, especially to school. Whenever I went outdoors, I had to have a large sun hat to hide my bald head from the rest of the world. People would pass me by and stare at me. I felt as if they were pitying me and I really did not want that. Many of my friends and relatives claimed that I looked "cute". This may well have been true but it still did not stop my little heart from aching inside. I also had my Dad's incessant teasing to cope with. But really, I enjoyed it, because it made me feel happy even though I was sad, if you know what I mean. His pet name for me was "peanut head". Can you believe it?

I can recall going out shopping, to the park or to some event, and staring at the pretty little girls wearing their long hair in braids or plaits and the ones that had short hair wore their hair with clips or hair bands. Did they realise how lucky they were to have hair? I don't suppose they even thought about it. Here was I admiring them and they were so carefree and unaware of what was going on around them. Yes, all my beautiful soft curls had gone! How long would it take for all of it to grow back? I was informed by the doctors that it might not grow back the same colour and that it might be a different texture. So: how about a colourful wig? By August 1995, three months after my diagnosis and treatment when I had lost all my hair, my parents decided we should all have a holiday to restore some sort of normality to life and give us a chance to reflect and be positive about the future. Hence, we ended up in Butlin's holiday camp. While walking around the complex one day, Dad spotted a bright blue dazzling wig which

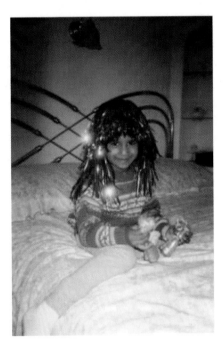

Fig. 20.   Janine with a colourful wig. Age, nearly 5.

he thought would be most appropriate fun (?) for me. I don't know how appropriate it really was but I felt like a film star.

School Life

School life for me was going to be so much more different than that of any other young child. The start of school life nearly did not happen for me. I was due to start school in the September of 1995. However, I was diagnosed with leukaemia in May 1995. What a way to start the most important part of your life!

When I actually did manage to get to school in that September, I was very apprehensive and scared. Any child's first day at school is daunting enough but I would be different from anyone else in the class: I was a girl with no hair. So I would not fit into either the girls or the boys group, or so I felt. I would be missing quite a lot of school initially so everyone else would have already made friends and I would have to fit into any group as best as I could. The first day of primary school was even harder. Gripping both my parents' hands, I entered into the multi-purpose room of St Stephen's Primary School in Welling, Kent. I looked around the room at all the other children. Why can't I be like them, I thought silently? Why? Deep in my own thoughts, I had not realised I was standing next to another girl my age. Like me, her family originated from Goa in India. She looked up at me and grinned. "I'm Nicole. What's your name?" she asked, playing with the hem of her new pinafore. I returned her friendly smile, "My name is Janine." Both mine and Nicole's parents exchanged smiles as well and began to chat immediately. Shyly, she held my hand and led me over to talk to some of the other children that were going to be in our class. Next, the reception teachers entered the room and introduced themselves. Miss Newton, my reception teacher, was extremely friendly and made everyone feel welcome. School was not so bad after all.

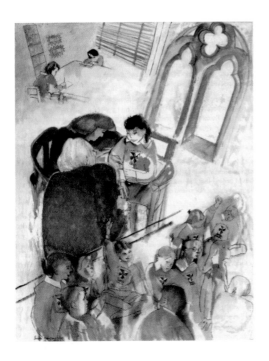

'*Back to School*' by Susan Macfarlane.

"*A very normal child who seemed at ease with the treatment and happy to talk about it to us all. I very much enjoyed the natural curiosity of many of the children as to what I could possibly be doing.*" A painting depicting medical treatment as part of normal life. The main part shows a nurse taking blood from a child. This is surrounded by scenes of everyday school activity. In one, Annie, the child, is shown working at a table. The Gothic window in the background helps identify the setting as a classroom. A scene at the bottom of the composition shows her class during a question session in which each class member was encouraged to relate personal experiences of hospital. Oil on Canvas. 91 × 71 cm. (Courtesy of Euan and Angus Mackay and Dr Geoffrey Farrer-Brown).

I did have highs and lows at school with the boys taking my sun hat off my head and running off with it for a joke. Except, to me, it was not so funny and it was another thing I had to cope with. However, once the teacher found out about it she sat the children down and explained to them the seriousness of what they were doing and it soon stopped. On the other hand, the majority of the children and teachers at school were extremely supportive and made me feel as if I was one of them, just a normal girl attending reception class at primary school. That's all I wanted to be: just normal.

Then came the worst scenario of all for me. I had a bone infection in my foot which meant I could not walk on it for a while. I would have to sit in a buggy and be pushed around in it like a little baby. Well, I can tell you I was less than impressed with this. First of all, I had a bald head and now I had to be pushed around in a buggy at school. I really felt like a little baby now. Anyway, what did everyone else care, it was me that would be ridiculed. However, I soon learnt it was not going to be like that at all. St Stephen's had always been most accommodating to me. They said they would like me to attend school even if it meant being pushed around in a buggy. They said they would make arrangements with the staff and children to care for me fully while I was at school. I can remember the older girls in Years 5 and 6, pushing me around the library, the playground or the different classrooms. I think I felt a little bit odd sitting in a buggy at my age. I mean, I had seen various children walking with crutches due to sprained or broken ankles, but none in buggies! On the other hand, I felt like a local celebrity, what with people wheeling me up to the lunch queue and holding my tray for me! It can't have been all that bad. So that was a hurdle that we all overcame.

Overall, my school life was made much easier for me during my illness due to the care, help and support that I received from St Stephen's School. My particular appreciation goes to my head-teacher, Mrs Masterson and the School Secretary, Mrs Smith for their endless help in sorting out situations for me which would enable me to remain in school during my illness. I could not have wished for a more caring and nurturing environment. Looking back now, I know they took a lot of pressure off my parents in terms of my education and well being while at school. I could never thank them enough. I feel it was this positive learning environment which has enabled me to do so well during my schooling throughout the years.

As for my primary education, I was definitely not "hard done by", especially at GOSH. With a whole classroom and a teacher all to myself, I learnt a great deal. I felt privileged not having to share the teacher's attention with thirty other children! I guess that it was these one-to-ones sessions that really helped me compensate for the two years of schooling that I was to miss out on. The infamous "Scaredy Cat" game is still vivid in my mind. It used to drive my parents absolutely crazy, but it kept me entertained for hours, much to my Mum and Dad's dismay! GOSH could be likened to a glorified hotel, packed with games and toys, just for me. When I was not in the open bays, I had my own private room with a television. Can you believe it? In fact, I can even recall begging my Dad to play on the *Mario Brothers* video game with me everyday. At the time, I felt as if I had the best of everything. However, this all came at a very high price of having leukaemia. That is the sharp reality of it all.

I enjoyed attending the hospital schools at Queen Mary's and GOSH. It gave me an opportunity to meet other children, which was a real joy for me because I was normally in an isolated room in a ward due to my low resistance to infections. It was also an opportunity for me to socialise with children of varying ages. Some people might think it strange that I wanted to mix with other children in a hospital ward. However, for me at that stage, it was the only opportunity to talk about child-like things. At least by doing this, I felt somewhat normal.

As you can imagine, I missed quite a lot of those first few years at school due to my treatment. Looking back on the situation, I do not know how I would have coped with all that today. Perhaps it was better that I had to endure this as a very young child.

Second Home

While receiving treatment, Queen Mary's and GOSH became my second homes. The one distinction between the two hospitals was that I felt more at home at GOSH purely for the fact that I was not so different from anyone else. We all looked much the same with our bald heads, walking round the hospital corridors with our mobile drips. I sometimes imagined that we were like aliens on another planet. I think by fantasizing, it helped me to overcome the fact that we had to cope with being bald. I can vividly remember the first day I entered the children's ward at GOSH. Giraffe Ward, it was called. As I walked, hand in hand with both my parents, I saw painted giraffe tiles on the walls of the corridors. They were so captivating for a child of my age. Children's paintings (from the ward) were also hung around the windows. In fact, even now, when I visit the Elephant Day Care Centre and see those paintings and the children, I still get chills up and down my spine. I was one of those children, once. Anyway, I soon found myself with lots of new friends at the hospital, both children and nursing staff alike. Without me even knowing it, they became an integral part of my life.

I could not want for anything more at GOSH. I had my own room with a television and a video and a separate bathroom. Even my Mum and Dad had their own bed in my room. The hospital certainly created that feeling of being at home as best as they could. There was even a separate TV and play room with hundreds of toys. I remember the nurses, doctors and consultants being so friendly and kind. However, the comforts at GOSH still did not make up for the fact that I would endure some pretty awful treatment with terrible side effects which would make me feel very unwell.

By day, I would be fed intravenous chemotherapy drugs, it seemed like an endless cocktail of drugs being administered to me. Then I would need some more drugs to help me cope with the side effects such as nausea and vomiting. Then I had to have the normal blood tests, blood and platelet transfusions when my blood counts were very low. Besides this, I had to encounter numerous liver function tests to check that my liver was not being damaged; heart echoes to check that my heart was not being damaged, and the story goes on.

I remember being woken up in the middle of the night by two nurses who would have to change my drip. They would wear these awful looking glasses and these big plastic gloves to protect themselves from these lethal chemotherapy drugs they were administering into me.

I was not allowed many visitors here as the treatment I was having was quite strong and it did make me feel very unwell. However, I do remember spending some really good quality time with my Mum and Dad. Obviously, this was to the detriment of my baby sister Kirsten. I would say to my Mum "does Kirsten miss you?" Mum would be polite and say "course she does, but she has lots of lovely people to look after her".

My Best Friends: Freddie and the Infamous Emla Cream

Those two years of treatment were possibly the worst two years of my life. As the chemotherapy drugs were destroying most of my white blood cells, I was left with little resistance to infections such as the common cold and chicken pox. So, as well as going into hospital for my regular blocks of treatment, I was frequently in hospital with dangerously high temperatures and fever. My body just did not have the strength to fight these infections. It reached such a ridiculous point that if any child in my class had chicken pox, their parents would have to alert the teachers, so I could be taken out of school, to avoid any risk of infection.

I had one best friend with me throughout my two years of treatment and that was Freddie, my Hickman line. He was my saving grace. Initially, when he was inserted into my chest cavity wall, it was the first operation I had been through with a general anaesthetic. I could feel the tension on my parents' faces as I was finally wheeled off to have the line inserted into me. I woke up from this operation bewildered and not knowing what to expect. Anybody might have thought I had grown an extra arm! But in all seriousness, this served as a great comfort throughout my treatment. To me, Freddie basically meant two things. No constant needles and no pain. What a star Freddie was, or so I thought at the time. Yes, Freddie took the pain each time I received chemotherapy treatment or had a blood test. However, he also served as a great nuisance. He followed me around everywhere I went. I guess that was probably likely, since the darn thing was attached to my chest for two years! I can recall having to tape it up when I went for a bath every night and then I would let it hang down lose, like a long snake, when I was finished. I had these terrible nightmares that as I was playing with my friends one day they would yank it out of my chest by mistake. However, I need not have worried as it was firmly embedded inside me. It was an emotional occasion when Freddie was removed from me after the two years of treatment. Of course I felt elated but then I felt a sort of sadness come over me. After all, he had been through all the good and bad times with me and now we were going to part ways.

I would also like to share my memories of the infamous emla cream. Throughout my treatment, emla cream became my second best friend. It was always there to numb any part of my body before the needle was inserted into my skin. Without it, I would have had a lot of pain everytime I had to have a needle inserted into me and considering the amount of needles I had to have, this would have

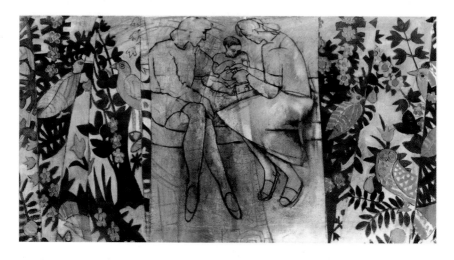

'*The Hickman Line*' by Susan Macfarlane.
"*An intimate scene glimpsed between curtains showing a nurse and mother tending a small child who is receiving an infusion of drugs.*" This is given through a Hickman line, or central venous catheter (a thin flexible multi-channel plastic tube inserted under the skin of the chest into a large vein just above the collar bone), which allows the easy administration of intravenous drugs and the taking of blood samples. Oil on Canvas. 46 × 86 cm. (Courtesy of Euan and Angus Mackay and Dr Geoffrey Farrer-Brown).

meant pain frequently. So once again I have to thank the person that invented emla cream. It was a blessing in disguise for me. I am sure it is just so for every other child who suffers from leukaemia and has to go through what I had to endure.

Mum, Dad and Hospital Life

Throughout my diagnosis and treatment, I can recall that my Mum and Dad were always there by my side. No matter how bad things were, they were always there for me. There were constant words of encouragement and praise to help me to stay positive. Obviously, being so young at the time, you do not realise what sort of pain and suffering they were going through. They had to cope with an immense amount of pressure. They had to be with me, attend to work situations, sort out home life and care for my baby sister, Kirsten. It is only now that I realise the full impact of what leukaemia can have on family life. You do not actually have a life because you are not able to do the everyday normal things that a family does. Your life revolves around treatments and hospitals; there is nothing else you can fit in.

I can recall my Mum, in particular, sitting by my bedside day and night. Mum had to give up work to look after me. I can specifically remember all the magazines and toys she used to buy for me or bring to me in hospital. Whenever I felt lonely or bored, she would pick up my colouring pencils and draw or colour with me to keep me occupied. Even late at night when I could not sleep due to the discomfort of the drip attached to my arm, she would always talk, in her gentle, soft voice to me. She would always try and reassure me that everything would be alright. There was something about the way she used to talk to me that helped me to relax and remain calm. Whether it was holding my hand during an injection or completing a crossword puzzle with me, she was always there for me. I have to give credit to my Dad also. He worked odd hours but after work, and no matter where he had been, he would always be there for me. It did not matter how hard or tiring it was, he would not let me down. I can look back on it now and say that without my Mum and Dad's positive attitude to the leukaemia, I would not have been able to come through it.

Cocktails, Jelly and Drugs

During the protocol, a drug called daunorubicin was frequently administered to me, as one of the main drugs. At first, I used to think that it was some type of fruit juice, like Rubicon. Little did I know that it was anything but a cocktail. I now understand that it was this particular drug that caused my hair loss. As well as this, it appeared to have some risks to my heart. I recall the consultant saying to my parents that there was a possibility of vegetation on my heart valves.

Due to this risk, I was carted off annually to receive a heart echo, which would determine if any major damage had occurred. I used to be extremely suspicious when I entered that dark, black room, with both of my parents. One can say that I was fascinated with all the monitors and the different noises they made. The next minute, I was laid down flat on the bed, with about a million stickers all over my chest. Then, the worst part came. That cold, slimy, disgusting saline jelly. All over my body. It was absolutely everywhere. I can remember trying to shut my eyes as tight as possible trying to forget the fact that a cold, mucus-like substance was being spread, like marmalade, on my chest. Although I was not really allowed to turn my head around to look at the monitor, I took "sneaky peeks" at the screen, as I was so intrigued to see what was going on inside my body. It was like watching a fish aquarium. Many coloured dots just filled the screen — they were completely mesmerising to me. In addition to this, every so often, the cardiologist would switch on the sound and I would be able to hear my heart beating viciously. However, as the chemotherapy drugs have left lasting effects on my heart, it is still compulsory to receive these heart echoes, to check any backflow of blood through the valves. At least now I only have to be examined every five years, instead of yearly. I have to say, honestly, that even though I am not a first timer with these heart echoes, I still feel anxious and sick before I enter that dark room. Maybe that is just the way I am.

My parents were soon told by Dr Rassam that I had been entered for the UKALL 11 trials. What on earth did this mean? My parents, almost as confused as me, did not have a single clue about what this was. Would there be disadvantages? Would there be any advantages? More questions. Well, in simple terms, it meant that I had been entered for a three-block treatment, in which the dosage of chemotherapy drugs administered to me was to be more intense than usual. Not that difficult to understand, right? My parents had been told that I had been randomly chosen for a particular "arm" of this trial and due to this, I would have to receive a high dose of methotrexate and mercaptopurine (a type of maintenance treatment). Do not ask me how I remembered the name of these drugs as a young child. Perhaps it was because they were drummed into my head every single day for those two years of treatment. Anyway, I can recall that after every block of treatment I received, I took the maintenance drugs. It was like a routine procedure. Imagine this. A regular four-year-old brushes her teeth, eats breakfast and then goes to school every morning. For me, it was chemotherapy five days a week for two years. Still, I did not think anything of it at the time. Not unfair. Not cruel. Just an everyday kind of thing.

After each block of treatment, I can remember having to take some drugs orally. Yes, tablets also became regularity in my life. God, it is no wonder I can remember the name of all those drugs. I had to take them every single day! Still, I guess anything was better than having to go to hospital. While in hospital, I can remember so many people coming in and out to visit me. Relatives, doctors, nurses, you just name it. In particular, my grandparents were frequent visitors. All the sweets, chocolates, fruit and Robinson's Orange squash were enough to fill up the whole hospital room! Obviously, they did not understand about leukaemia as much as my parents did, but they did, however, realise the severity of the situation. I had cancer. Even though I have to give credit to the chemotherapy, my grandparents' love and affection for me definitely gave me the strength and courage I needed at a time of such hardship. Other visitors included a social worker, who guided my parents on how to care for me after the treatment and several medical professionals, who tended to me on a daily basis. I felt as if I had met the whole world after those two years.

"One Step Forward, Two Steps Back"

One can look at fighting leukaemia as a race for life. However, as I came into the finishing stages of this race to have Freddie, my Hickman line removed, I had to encounter yet another hurdle. What we all saw as the light at the end of the tunnel now seemed like miles away. Disaster struck yet again. I had begun to complain about a terrible pain in my left foot. It turned out that I had developed an infection in that foot. So, it was back again to the hospital. The local hospital could not make a diagnosis. Once again, I had to endure test after test. Finally, GOSH said that they would remove my Hickman line, which was due to be taken out at this point, and at the same time, they would take a biopsy of the foot. Two for the price of one. It really was not very funny at the time but I suppose I can look back on it now and smile about it a little. Anyway, it turned out that I had osteomyelitis, a bone infection, which made an area of my foot extremely painful to walk on. So once again, I was in hospital. I thought to myself how unlucky I was at that time.

Winning the Race

By April 1997, we had reached that light at the end of the tunnel. We had finally arrived at the last hurdle, the end of treatment, and could not wait to take that leap forward. However, even at this point, there were still doubts in my mind. I had to have Freddie, my Hickman line removed, but now I had the additional problem with my foot. Till I went into surgery and had a biopsy and till the results were confirmed, I still had to wait. I could not get over excited as my whole world might collapse again. I felt I could not be too positive even at this stage. As I came out of theatre, after having my Hickman line removed, I can remember seeing Freddie, lying detached, on a small tray, beside my hospital bed. In fact, I still keep him as a memento in a box with all my other treasured belongings.

I just wanted to be normal again. What would it feel like not having injections, treatment, infections and the rest of it? Would I even know how to act normal? For two years, I had to follow a hospital-based routine and now I had to face the prospect of living a normal childhood. That is if leukaemia did not return. This was always in the back of my mind. Obviously, I still had to receive regular blood tests and routine check-ups at the local hospital and at GOSH. However, I guess anything was better than finding myself attached to a drip, sitting in some hospital bed, and sulking because I felt so unwell at times.

I must say the highlight of the end of my treatment was when my parents, accompanied by my grandparents, took me to Lourdes, a place of pilgrimage for Roman Catholics and as a thanksgiving to God for helping me to come through my treatment with a positive outcome. Most of the friends I made while at both hospitals talked about visiting Disneyland in Florida. It had always been a dream for my grandparents to take me to Lourdes, in thanksgiving for the return of my good health. Since I had just come out of hospital from my foot infection and biopsy, I was unable to walk so I had to be pushed around in a buggy. I can honestly say that visiting Lourdes was a very peaceful and soothing experience for me and my family. It was like the calm after the storm. I think it gave all of us time to reflect on the past two years, the trials and tribulations, the highs and the lows, and the joy and sadness as events unfolded. All of us were always on the edge because we could not foresee what was to befall us.

While in Lourdes, I can remember my whole family visiting Our Lady's grotto everyday. I took great pleasure in lighting candles that were twice the size of myself. Now, I do not know whether any of you believe in miracles, but even I do not think I did until this moment that I am now going tell you about. Everyday that I was in Lourdes, I bathed my painful foot in the holy water from the springs originating from the grotto (these springs were started by St Bernadette). When we all arrived back at London Gatwick Airport, I realised that my foot was no longer painful and I did not have a limp. First of all, I thought I was imagining it. However, I then strode around in my LA Gear trainers which gave me great pleasure as they were the ones that lighted up when you walked on them. Miracle or not, I was elated that I could walk again. So that was one of the last hurdles I would have to conquer and what a relief it was. My Mum and Dad kept telling me we were winning the fight.

Sometimes, I feel as though I do not realise what a tough, gruelling and testing time I suffered. I had more injections and blood tests than I could count, I had missed out on most of two years of schooling and lost all of my hair, just to mention a few downsides. In my honest opinion, I believe that I was stronger as a young child than I am now. "The little battler," was what my parents used to call me, and in some respects, I suppose they were right. Even though I was so young, there must have been some voice of strength at the back of my brain urging me not to give up and let the leukaemia win.

Looking Forward

After my gruelling two years of treatment, I certainly was looking forward to the rest of my life. Who can say what the future holds for us but I am going to do my utmost to enjoy life to the best of my ability.

As you can imagine, having experienced leukaemia has left quite an imprint on my life. Besides the emotional side of having the illness, you also have to deal with the physical scars. Everytime I go for a shower and look at my chest, there is an ugly scar to remind me about the time Freddie was attached to me. But, I guess I just have to live with that. Not a day goes by without me thinking of what I had to go through as a child. However, looking back on it, I am glad that I had leukaemia when I was only a child. Since I was so young, I did not really understand a lot of what was going on and my parents made the decisions for me. It was a lot easier that way.

Even after my two years of treatment I was not free from hospital visits as I had to attend the local hospital for tests to ensure the disease was not returning. In addition, I had to attend the follow-up clinic at GOSH so that they could monitor my progress in relation to the UKALL 11 trial that I was part of. This involved me in undergoing heart echoes and scans to ensure that the lethal cocktail of drugs had not damaged my liver or heart. The hospital also had to monitor my learning abilities as one of the drugs, daunorubicin, could have affected my mental skills. I am very pleased to say that none of the drugs seemed to have had any such effect. I have been attending Newstead Wood School for Girls since 11 years of age, this being one of the top ten secondary schools in the UK. In my opinion, Newstead is a school full of opportunity. It has inspired me and taught me that you can achieve success if you work hard at it. Whilst at the school, I tried to enlighten my classmates about leukaemia. I had the opportunity to do this when we were asked to give a talk on any particular subject. Well, this was my chance. I gave everyone a general background into the causes of leukaemia, my own positive experience of the illness and then I talked about my good friend Brendan, who died of leukaemia at the age of twelve. To my astonishment, I received a standing ovation from the class, which I must say overwhelmed me slightly. Even though I felt it important to share my experience with others, they will never really know my true experience with leukaemia. I don't think anyone will.

Looking back now from the age of four to the present day, I know that having leukaemia has made me realise now that life is such a very precious gift which few people realise. It is not until you are really ill with some illness like leukaemia that you appreciate how wonderful life is. Sometimes when I sit and look back, I feel resentful because I feel that having the leukaemia has robbed me of my childhood and it is something I will never ever be able to experience again. I have lost that part of my life forever. I feel sad when my friends talk about their childhood experiences because all I can talk about is hospitals, treatments and feeling unwell. When I was feeling really sad and despondent at times, I remember I would ask my Mum why God had given me this illness to bear as opposed to any other children. Being religious as well as tactful, my Mum would always give me the same answer, "The only reason God gave you leukaemia, Janine, is because he knows you have the strength to fight it." I believed her then, as I do now.

The only way that I can overcome these feelings is by turning my illness into something positive. You may well ask how one can do that. However, even though it brought me and my family tremendous times of suffering, hardship and despair, it taught me to have hope. It served as a learning curve for me and it taught me about the presence of personal will and strength to overcome not only the illness but problems in other aspects of life. It has made me more eager to learn about the subject now that I am much older and capable of understanding the complexities of the disease. When I was diagnosed, I had about a 67% chance of survival. As a child, I did not understand what "sixty-seven percent" actually meant. Nevertheless, I now know that it was a pretty good survival rate. Now, due to ongoing research and major advances in science, technology and medicine in the study of leukaemia, the survival rates for children are much higher.

My motto in life is that if you can beat leukaemia, then you can conquer anything that life has to throw your way. Through my own experiences of the illness, I would like to give others encouragement to face what they have to bear with strength and a positive attitude of mind. And I would say to them you can beat this illness if you stay positive. My final message to anyone of any age who has been diagnosed with leukaemia, is to stay positive and tackle each hurdle as it arises. Do not confront the problems before they arise or you will not be able to handle the pressures which the leukaemia brings along with it. It just goes to show that even when you have had to encounter such a terrible illness like leukaemia, you can still achieve your goals in life. I hope that I am a living proof of that.

A FAMILY'S JOURNEY: THE MOTHER

Delena Fernandes

As a parent of two young children, Janine aged four and Kirsten aged just six months old at the time, you wake up everyday wondering what challenges and joy you will experience that day. However, no one prepares you for the worst day of your life. This will be the day when everything changes and there is no turning back. As the cliché says "life will never be the same again". Believe me, it rings so true.

How could a parent not know that their child was so ill? This is the harsh reality we had to face when Janine was diagnosed with leukaemia. How could we, as parents, let her become so ill and not even be aware of it? There were no extreme symptoms such as weight loss, loss of appetite, bruising, or so we thought. However, recalling all the symptoms Janine did have at the time and prior to the diagnosis, it was so obvious, but what parent succumbs to these sorts of thoughts? In the lead up to Janine's diagnosis, she had recurrent infections, mostly colds, flu-like symptoms and earaches with high temperature. These necessitated repeated visits to the GP. Janine had a tummyache at preschool a week before she was diagnosed and a bad nose bleed at her friend's birthday party. She did have bruises on her leg but not an excessive amount that you would be concerned about. One day when I asked her to fetch a pillow from upstairs for me, she explained that she was too tired to go and get it for me. We put this down to pure laziness.

It was quite by chance that we discovered Janine was seriously ill. It was her sister Kirsten's check up with the health visitor and I took Janine along with me. The health visitor carried out the normal checks for Kirsten, and by pure luck or coincidence, I asked her to have a look at Janine for me. I do not know why I did it as I was not particularly concerned about her health at that time. The health visitor weighed Janine and asked to see the inside of her bottom eyelid and then took a look at her tongue and her skin colouration. Without hesitation, she asked me to take Janine to the doctor immediately. I asked her if there was a problem. She obviously thought there was but was not prepared to tell me at that stage and I assumed that, anyway, she could not be certain of any diagnosis. I trusted her judgement as she had been Janine's health visitor from the time she was born. Later on, I found out from her that she had started her training as a doctor but gave up and became a health visitor instead. What a godsend she was! I promised her I would make an appointment at the doctor's surgery that evening. When I left the health clinic, I just knew something was seriously wrong with Janine. You could call it a mother's intuition. I wanted to cry but I did not want to upset the girls. So I put on a brave face and walked home.

Immediately, I got home and rang my husband. He asked me how I had got on with Kirsten at the clinic. I can remember those words which haunt me everytime I talk about Janine's leukaemia; I said, "Don't worry about Kirsten. We need to be worried about Janine".

What follows is a series of events which I can remember as if they happened yesterday. Does one ever forget how it all started? I took Janine to the doctor's surgery and explained to him why I was there. He said we needed to send Janine for a blood test the following morning. I remember asking him if I should be concerned. He obviously did not want to worry me unnecessarily and kept saying to me that we should wait until we get the blood results. I did not even ask him specifically what he was checking for. I think at this point again, I began worrying a lot more. I felt he was hiding some information from me. The following day, we took Janine for her blood test in the morning. Nervous, worried and anxious, we pulled up outside Queen Mary's Hospital in Sidcup. Little did we know at that time this would be like our second home for the next two years. We got the blood test done and went back home. It was a very peculiar day. My in-laws and a close relative were at home with us. I remember it being a lovely hot sunny day but there was this cloud hanging over us. I could not motivate myself to do anything until I knew for certain what exactly was wrong with Janine.

It was around five o'clock in the evening and I remember it so vividly. I was in the kitchen and then the doorbell rang. I went to the front door and it was our local doctor, Dr Banerjee, who only lived a few doors away from us. For some reason I walked into the kitchen and he followed me. He said Janine had been diagnosed with leukaemia and that we needed to take her to see a consultant at Queen Mary's Hospital, first thing the next morning. First of all, I did not know what leukaemia was. I kept telling him to wait for my husband to come downstairs and then explain to both of us, but he just kept talking to me and I was not listening to him. I kept asking him over and over again if he was sure and could there be a possibility that a mistake had been made. He replied "no". At this point, I was hysterical. I was crying and shouting and shaking. I just could not take all this on board in such a short space of time. At this point, I do not think I had any energy left in me; it seemed to have been drained away from my body. I felt numb. What was I supposed to do next? This was my little girl with cancer in her body eating away inside her. One thing I was grateful for was that she was not suffering any pain at this point, and that was what really mattered to me at this stage. Other things we would have to deal with as they came our way.

I put on my brave, mummy face and asked Janine what sort of a treat did she want for dinner. She replied "Macdonald's please". From the time the doctor visited to give us the bad news to approximately an hour later, we had phone call after phone call from friends and relatives offering us support and help in anyway they could. This was the start of many years of wonderful support from our friends and family, which we could not have done without. They were our rock in moments of sadness, despair and frustration. The rest of that evening was somewhat a blur. I can recall friends coming through the front door and hugging and comforting us. They also cried with us. I was exhausted by the end of the day and felt weary, depressed and sad. However, I was told by everyone that I should not cry in front of her, so I didn't. They said I needed to be strong for her sake.

My husband and I slept with Janine that night. We snuggled her in the middle of us. Both of us could not sleep that night. I kept saying to my husband "what if we lose her?", "what if she dies?", "what are we going to do without her?" I kept looking at her and thinking she was my baby and she was beautiful but I did not know what was going to happen to her at that point. I started getting angry, thinking how could this disease have got hold of her. She was too young to be ill. And at this point, there was nothing me or my husband could do to help her to get better. As a parent, you feel you have a responsibility to keep your children safe from harm but we were not capable of doing that now. We felt we had let her down badly. I kept asking Janine, "Are you in any pain?" I got a response, "No mummy." But even then, I did not believe her. Was she trying to hide her pain from me so that I would not be upset?

That night went so slowly, neither my husband nor I slept at all. We wanted the night to be over as quickly as possible because we wanted to know Janine's chances of survival. At this stage, all we knew about leukaemia was that it was cancer of the blood. That was the total depth of our knowledge. It was probably a good thing at that stage as we would have been even more worried that night.

On our way to the hospital that morning, our heads were full of negative thoughts because of the lack of knowledge of the disease. I think at that stage, questions such as how long have we still got with her and how much pain would she have to endure before the inevitable happens, kept cropping into our heads. It was probably not that long that we had to sit in the waiting room of the haematology department for the consultant to see us, but for us, it felt like we had been waiting forever. I kept watching everyone who entered and I kept telling myself: they are just coming in for a blood test and we have to face this terrible meeting with the consultant to confirm an awful diagnosis for our child. In my mind, all these people in the waiting room were so lucky, but did they realise it?

We were escorted into the consultant's room and sat down. He was a man of small stature but very friendly, Dr Saad Rassam. He sat us down and explained that Janine had leukaemia and what, in essence, this disease was. He explained that there were two types of leukaemia and that if you could have the better type then this was it. Dr Rassam said Janine had acute lymphoblastic leukaemia (or ALL). At that time, it did not matter to me what type she had because to me she had this incurable disease, at least that is what I thought. Dr Rassam explained that there were several factors in her favour. He said she was a girl and because of the makeup of their bodies they stood a better chance of survival. Her age was also a big factor in her prognosis. He then went on to explain that she had a 70 percent chance of survival. He kept talking to us but I do not know how much of it I was actually taking in. It was all too much in a short space of time. What amazed us was that we did not realise how ill Janine already was at this stage. Dr Rassam explained that Janine was quite ill, with an infection and her blood count was low. We were told that she would have to be taken straight from the consulting room into a ward and be treated as quickly as possible. There were so many questions we needed to ask at that stage but we just could not think of any of them. That is apart from one question. We told Dr Rassam that we wanted the best for Janine and that we would go to a private hospital if it meant that she would get better treatment there. We were aware that the NHS had problems with funding and would sometimes not be able to offer the best and new treatments due to financial constraints. Dr Rassam reassured us that he would be looking after her and would offer her the best type of treatment to optimise her chances of survival. He also mentioned that for her to be treated privately, we would need around £300,000 to fund her treatment for the next two years. We took some comfort from his words. The burden was slightly lifted from us in so far as we had now handed Janine's care to a professional. There was nothing more we could do but wait. I felt that at least Janine was in very capable hands now and we had to let the professionals get on with their job. For me, it was a turning point because I did not realise Janine was so ill. Fortunately, now there was someone who would take good care of her. So for me, that was a fulfilment of responsibility, to a degree anyway.

Diagnosis

Going straight from the consulting room to the ward with Janine did not leave me with any time to ponder and think about anything. Two wonderful Irish nurses, Jane and Carol, were ready and waiting for us in a room in Lamorbey Ward. They explained that Janine would have to be in a room on her own due to the risk of infection. They took us into the room and then went off to get some equipment. In the meantime, I just looked around the room and felt scared. My head was spinning round and round. At this point, your whole life is turned upside down. You feel as if the whole world is closing in on you and there is no escape. You, as the parent, have to face up to the reality and what is to follow. However, you are left feeling numb inside and so frightened and scared of the consequences. The stark reality is that your child could die. At this stage, I just wanted to know what the outcome of all the treatments would be but I did not want to go through the whole process to find out. I was frightened, scared, feeling lost and very alone even though there were friends and family around me. I felt that this was something I had to deal with myself and even though I could talk to people, they really did not understand what I was going through because they had not experienced it themselves.

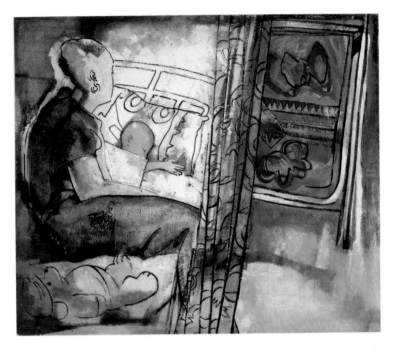

'*Sleeping It Off*' by Susan Macfarlane.
This shows the same child painted after the lumbar puncture. "*It seemed that this small person was still away with the butterflies in the colourful mural.*" The nurse watches tenderly. Nurses on this children's ward wear a special casual uniform to help the children feel more at ease. Oil on Canvas. 66 × 76.5 cm. (Courtesy of Euan and Angus Mackay and Dr Geoffrey Farrer-Brown). This image also used on the book cover.

Looking back now, I did not realise how selfish I was being at the time. It was Janine who was ill but I had never really considered how she might be feeling. I cannot remember talking to her at this point and saying to her that she had leukaemia and telling her what it was in simplistic terms or even what treatment she would have to endure. Maybe it was too painful for me then as I was still getting to grips with the diagnosis myself. But even so, I should have talked to her about it. She must have felt scared, upset and unsettled. One minute her life was as normal as any four and a half year old, and all of a sudden it was doctors, blood tests and hospitals. However, Carol and Jane became our guardian angels. They put us all at ease. They sat Janine on the bed, got her a doll and explained what they would be doing to her. They asked her if she had any questions. I think she was so bewildered then that she just sat on the bed and nodded. Both the nurses then asked us if we knew what was going on and we just shook our heads. They said they would see to Janine first and then sit down with us and explain to us all they could. As promised, Jane sat down with a piece of paper and pencil in hand and wrote down all the chemotherapy drugs that would be administered to Janine. She also explained what the purpose of the drugs was and what possible side effects existed. I was so in awe of Jane at this point because I felt lost, not really knowing anything and she took the time and trouble in her busy schedule to sit down with me and my husband to explain this all to us. Being a staunch Roman Catholic, I felt that she had been given the task by God to take the time and trouble to sit with me and my husband to explain things to us in simple terminology. Whether this was right or wrong, I do not know, but that is how I felt at that time.

Guilt and Uncertainty

Throughout all this early phase of Janine's leukaemia, many difficult questions kept popping into our heads. In particular, how could we as parents, entrusted with the care and protection of our children, not see the tell tale signs that Janine was so ill? We had obviously failed miserably as parents, or so we felt. Were we to blame in the first place for her leukaemia? Would she have inherited a leukaemia gene from one of us and, if so, was our other daughter at risk? We could get no clear or reassuring answers. And if it was not some inherited gene, what might be the cause? We knew that scientists hadn't yet solved this problem but we naturally looked at our own lifestyle. We never used to eat a great deal of processed foods but we did begin to think maybe it was something to do with the additives and preservatives that were added to the food that we might have eaten that had caused her illness. We certainly felt that the two pylons on either side of our road might well be to blame. We had read up on the dangers of

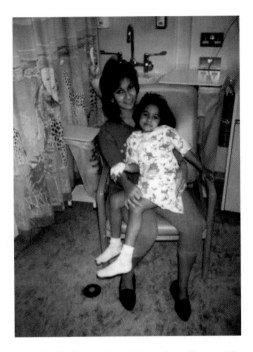

Fig. 21.   Photo of mum with Janine on first visit to Great Ormond Street Hospital and just before starting treatment.

pylons and felt that this was the main cause, especially to children with low immune systems. We felt particularly strongly about this because a boy who was aged five years old and who lived down the road from us was diagnosed with ALL exactly seven weeks prior to Janine's diagnosis. We also did our own research when we were at Great Ormond Street Hospital and ask parents if they lived near pylons or high voltage power cables. In every case, they replied yes. Still today, although we've been told it's very unlikely, we feel the cause lies with the pylon emissions.

Treatment: The Long Road

No one can prepare you for the gruelling treatment that your child needs to face when they have leukaemia. One common aspect of leukaemia is that before diagnosis, the child is normally ill in some way, with either an infection or a feeling of being unwell. But there is usually no obvious pain involved. It is only when you are faced with the two years of treatment that this situation changes. Your child has to endure countless blood transfusions, infections, lumbar punctures in the spine, bone marrow aspirates and chemotherapy which has to be administered by mouth or via injections in the thigh. Then, there is the emotional side of coping with your child while they go through this tough treatment regime. For a mother, this is like torture. I wished I had leukaemia instead of Janine. I kept asking myself, why did she have to undergo this when her life was just beginning? What a way to start your childhood. Not exactly the kind of memory you would like her to retain and later recall. Other children have wonderful memories of holidays with their families, visits to the seaside, walks in the park, bike rides, train journeys, trips to the zoo and the list just goes on. Our family life just came to a complete standstill, or so it seemed. We could not do any of this because of the fear of infection. Sometimes I would ask myself "Why does life have to be so cruel?" But I had to tell myself that this is just the way it is, grin and bear with it and just carry on for Janine's sake. Both my husband and myself felt that we needed to stay positive and confront this disease head on. After all, it was our daughter's life at stake and we had to do all that was physically and emotionally possible in order to help her to overcome this disease.

When Janine initially started her treatment at Queen Mary's Hospital, she had to have a cocktail of chemotherapy drugs which included vincristine, asparaginase, prednisolone and co-trimoxazole. Besides these drugs, she had to have countless number of blood transfusions, antibiotics for infections, platelet transfusions. In addition to all that, she had to have bone marrow aspirates and lumbar punctures to ascertain if the cancer had spread any further. I was very concerned about possible side effects and asked the doctors administering these medicines if they were all necessary. I could not imagine Janine's tiny little body withstanding such a toxic mixture of drugs. However, they replied bluntly but truthfully "It's essential for her survival". I could say no more.

Life for our family orbited in and around the hospital. Initially, Janine's treatment programme began at Queen Mary's Hospital but Dr Said Rassam advised us that Janine would receive shared care between Queen Mary's Hospital and GOSH. Arrangements were made for us to meet with Dr Ian Hann at GOSH to discuss her treatment programme there. We had many questions we needed to ask but Dr Hann obviously knew all our concerns and worries before we had even arrived there. By the time we left his consulting room, there was not one question unanswered. Dr Hann asked us if we would agree for her to be part of the UKALL 11 trial. He explained that the trial involved a two or three block treatment programme. The particular block of treatment that Janine would receive would be done on a random basis. We did wonder at that time if the two block treatment would be enough to kill all of the leukaemic cells. Then there was a dilemma with the three block treatment because it might have been too much for Janine's body to handle and would she be able to cope with the side effects? One of the objectives of this trial was to minimise possible late effects of treatment, in particular with respect to learning problems. We agreed to be part of the trial because we felt that if Janine had to go through chemotherapy treatment anyway, we could possibly help those who, unfortunately, would develop the disease in later years.

Our first day at GOSH was one I will never forget. As we made our way up to Giraffe Ward, we saw children looking so pale and gaunt with drips and various kinds of gadgets attached to them. We wondered if that would be Janine after her courses of strong chemotherapy drugs. But we were here now and we had to support Janine in any way we could. She was probably feeling quite daunted by the fact that she had to undergo all this treatment. I suspect we acted a little selfishly at that point and did not quite realise what Janine must have been going through. We were so wrapped up with our fears, worries and concerns that we ignored the fact that she too had feelings and anxieties, which she might have been afraid to share with us. Any fears or worries were alleviated for a little while anyway when the staff nurse took us to our room. She gave us a tour of the room and ward. She then took the time and trouble to explain what would happen next. Once again, we were in a strange environment, away from home and uncertain as to what was to follow. I remember unpacking our bags and thinking this would have to be home for us for the next five days so we better make it as comfortable as possible for Janine. She was surrounded by her toys, games and videos. I think she was all right at that point.

Janine then had to endure the placement of a Hickman catheter under the skin of her chest wall to enable the doctors and nurses to take blood samples as well as give her blood transfusions, platelets and chemotherapy drugs. This was to be a life-saving gadget for Janine, and probably for many children suffering with cancer and who need many courses of chemotherapy treatment. Janine had a Hickman line for a period of two years during the course of her treatment. Although both my husband and I knew that Janine had to have the line inserted, we also felt very anxious about it. We had concerns about infections that it might cause and the physical scars which would be with her throughout her life. We imagined that as a girl who would love dressing up in pretty clothes, she might feel restricted because they would show off her scar. Yet these were decisions based on the priority of saving her life and we tried to put off any negative thoughts about far less important issues in a possible future. My husband, Richard, decided if Janine had to have this hideous gadget inserted into her for a period of two years, then he needed to do something bold as well. So he took the step of giving up drinking for the next two years as a sort of parallel sacrifice!

The intensive treatment then began with side effects such as the nausea, mouth ulcers and weight loss. This was to be the start of many months of worry over test results, scans, heart echoes, etc. However, we felt we were quite lucky in one respect because there were children at GOSH who were much younger than Janine who did not have much of a chance of survival and some of them did actually die while we were there. It put everything in perspective for us. We felt we were the lucky ones, at that moment anyway.

Janine went through a gruelling regime of chemotherapy treatment consisting of five days at GOSH and then time spent at home to recover, although this often didn't happen. We would come back from GOSH so that Janine could recover at home but within a few days would be back again at the local hospital because Janine was suffering from an infection. I would sit and cry and then try to compose myself. This meant our daily routine would have to be altered again. We would have to make arrangements for Kirsten to be cared for by her grandparents and then I would have to pack all our things for yet another hospital stay. I cannot count the number of times we had to undergo this ritual. Once again, our family life was on hold.

Religious Belief: Challenges and Comfort

Religion has always played a large part in our lives and was crucial in helping us to cope with the ordeal of Janine's leukaemia. As a Roman Catholic, I believed that God would help us to overcome all the trials and tribulations over the coming months. Prayers and Masses were offered for Janine throughout the world by friends and family. Anyone who went on pilgrimages to various holy places like Lourdes would offer Masses and have candles lit for Janine. The first week I went to Mass after Janine's diagnosis was a very painful and distressing experience. I cried the whole of the Mass. It was hard to come to terms with the fact that God could have inflicted this terrible illness on our daughter who was so young. Then on the other hand, through my faith, I believed He must have done this, or allowed this, for a reason. Could it be to test our faith? That is what I chose to believe at that time because I could not think of it in any other way. I kept asking Him why did it happen to her, but in the same breath telling Him that I did not mean for any other child to be inflicted with this illness either. It was this faith which kept me strong through the many days, months and years of sadness, despair, disappointment and frustration of dealing with this illness. There are so many highs and lows and you just deal with each day as it comes. In reality, that is the only way you can deal with it. You want to be happy and confident when the treatment is going right but then you feel that could all change in a short space of time, plunging you into deep sadness again. No one can really help or reassure you at that point, not even your closest family or friends.

Some people might think it strange for us to still be dedicated to our religion when this disease was bestowed on Janine. Initially, as all parents are, we were totally distraught and we asked the normal questions such as "Why our poor Janine?" However, as the days went on, we found an inner strength to carry on and would pray everyday for a positive outcome.

I can recall the times I spent with Janine especially at GOSH. It was here in the night I found comfort in prayers. Once Janine was settled at night by the nurses, I would wait till she had fallen asleep. It was then my time. It was my time to cry, to be sad, and to feel the pain that I was experiencing. No one could tell me to stop upsetting Janine by crying or being sad. I didn't want to show the world how I felt. I would lie down on my sofa bed in the corner of Janine's room and I would pray intently. I would make a pact with God and tell Him that if He saved her then I would never ever forget Him. I would then begin my usual ritual and I would sob bitterly. I felt that this was my only way of releasing my anger and frustration at everything. I would cry and cry till I was worn out and I felt lifeless. It was a kind of ritual I guess, but if it helped me to get through the night and through the following day, then that is what I would do.

Friends and Family

Friends and family were marvellous right from the word go and they all rallied round. So many daily things needed to be taken care of but I do not think either my husband or myself had the energy or the ability to cope properly at that point. They asked if we needed assistance with daily chores such as shopping. Most importantly, our youngest daughter, Kirsten who was only eight months old at the time had to be taken care of. At this difficult time, we could not devote attention to her. All our energies were channelled into caring for Janine, a daughter we could lose at any stage. We wanted to spend every minute of everyday with her. It could only be that way, for now anyway.

We have to be eternally grateful to both sets of grandparents who were always there by our side and helped us through both the good and bad times. They took over the role of parents to Kirsten so that we could focus all our attention and energy wholly on Janine. Kirsten was not deprived of love or care at any point because of Janine's illness. In fact, she was probably thoroughly spoilt and that was a great weight off our minds. However, there was also a downside to this care, because we missed Kirsten's saying Mama and Dada, learning to walk, experiencing the beginnings of her first tooth appearing, and all the normal blossoming of childhood.

Looking Back, Looking Forward

After the two years of treatment, both my husband and myself were able to draw some comfort and relief and could reflect on what we had all been through. It had been an exhausting, depressing journey with some highs but mostly lows when you did not know what the future held. We desperately wanted to know what the eventual outcome would be but we could be given no guarantee. This was the hardest part for us to handle; watching Janine going through all this tough treatment, unsure if it would benefit her ultimately. We could only sit and wait. The next five years of our life, after the two years of treatment, were plagued with constant worry and doubts. "Would Janine stay in remission?" Of course, some children do not. But very fortunately, Janine has and is now thriving as a bright and vibrant 17 year old.

During our time spent at both hospitals, we met some very kind, compassionate and caring doctors, nurses and consultants, in particular Dr Said Rassam at Queen Mary's Hospital. From the moment of Janine's diagnosis to those awful first few days when we were in a complete state of shock not knowing how bad the leukaemia was till the test results came through, Dr Rassam was always there for us, finding time to sit down and explain to us the complexities of leukaemia in a way we could understand. He would speak to Janine in a very soothing and calm voice, helping to put her at ease. He was obviously well aware that what she had to face would be quite harrowing and daunting. Even the small touches were there as when he came in with a gift of Janine's favourite chocolates. We still refer to Dr Rassam as "our saviour" and we will always be eternally grateful to him. There were also the wonderful nurses at both hospitals who would take the time and trouble, even though they were extremely busy, to stop and sit down for a few minutes to have a chat with us which meant so much to us. I think they knew we were at breaking point sometimes and especially when Janine's blood counts were low and her liver function tests were not what they should have been and when she was feeling unwell with yet another infection. Their words of understanding and encouragement spurred us on.

When Janine was diagnosed with leukaemia, we did not even know what the word meant till the doctor explained it to us. For both of us, as parents of a child diagnosed with leukaemia, we had so little knowledge of the disease. It was like taking a two year course in the understanding and treatment of leukaemia. We had no knowledge of what treatments were available, which chemotherapy drugs were used for which purpose, the side effects of the drugs, and the maintenance treatment involved. However, after Janine completed her treatment at both hospitals, I think we felt positively knowledgeable and we could have possibly advised on some of the treatments available, what blood counts were deemed to be alright and at what point blood and platelet transfusions were needed. It was definitely a steep learning curve for both my husband and myself.

Janine's leukaemia was one stage of our life that is now completed. We have now moved on from that to a more positive phase, ready to face the world again and anything it may throw at us. It may be a cliché but Janine's leukaemia has given us a different, broader and more sensitive perspective on life. Previously, we were not aware of the suffering and hardships people with ill health can face. Now we are better equipped to sympathise with them. It has made us conscious of the fact that people with serious illnesses are not the only victims; their families have to suffer alongside them, even more so when children are involved. And though it might seem a strange thing to say, we are glad that Janine had her leukaemia when she was a child and not, say, as an infant or older teenager. The reasons are simple: firstly, she had a much better chance of survival and, secondly, she does not remember too much about the most grim aspects and was unaware at the time of how big a threat to life it was. This can now, given the eventual outcome, be a positive thing for her.

It is only now that we can face talking to Janine about her leukaemia and to write these stories of our journeys with the disease. She wants to know exactly what she went through and what were her emotions at the time. She can remember certain parts of her treatment but others are less distinct in her memory.

We are very proud that Janine managed to survive this terrible illness and has come out to be a strong person. Even when she was undergoing treatment and did manage to snatch a few days here and there at school, she always did really well. Years on, she managed to gain a place at Newstead Wood School for Girls, a school which is rated one of the top 10 schools in the UK. And, just as we write, Janine has received fantastic news: she achieved no fewer than 12 A* ratings in her GCSE examinations. Of course, we are immensely proud of such an achievement, especially as she did not attend school regularly for two years of her life. She has always worked to the best of her ability, demands perfection from herself and always wants to please her Mum and Dad. We often say to her that she needs to be happy and contented with herself and especially with what she has been through. She is a lovable, fun loving girl with many friends. She is also extremely loving and caring to her sister Kirsten, who she dotes on. I think Janine realises that Kirsten, too, has missed out on a lot of love and attention in her early childhood.

Like all parents, we want the very best for Janine and we hope that all her hopes and dreams do come true, and especially so because of the ordeal she has endured. Now is her time to enjoy her life to the full and we are confident she will do well in whatever career she decides to venture into. She certainly has the drive and determination. She is ambitious, career-wise, but also appreciates the simple, ordinary things in life like going out with friends and shopping. Her greatest wish to date is to be a bridesmaid to someone. So if there are any offers out there, please do not hesitate to contact her!

Both my husband and myself made a conscious decision to raise money for leukaemia research because we had gained so much from it. It was something positive we could do, something we could give back. Gary Lineker, the well known English soccer player whose own son George had leukaemia, had given his backing to the Leukaemia Research Fund Bike Ride in central London in order to raise money for leukaemia research. Through friends and family, we raised £1500 in sponsorship money for that event, which we were elated with. The whole family was invited to a presentation event where the highlight of our evening was meeting with Mr and Mrs Lineker.

No parent should have to watch their child suffer. However, should you be unlucky, like ourselves, in having a child that is diagnosed with leukaemia, then the best and only way forward is to look at it in a positive perspective. Today, with the advances in medical research, so many more children survive this terrible disease. And everyday, yet more new advances are being made. It is through the tiresome work of people such as Professor Mel Greaves, Dr Donald Pinkel, and many other researchers and clinicians that we should be indebted to. We certainly are very grateful to them for their pioneering work.

So, stay positive. Take a look at our own journey with Janine and you will see a very positive outcome is possible at the end of a long, stormy road.

GLOSSARY OF TERMS

ALL	Acute lymphoblastic leukaemia
AML	Acute myeloblastic leukaemia
AmoL	Acute monoblastic leukaemia
B cell lineage	A major subtype of "lymphoid" white blood cell involved in antibody synthesis in immune responses
Chromosomes	23 pairs of chromosomes in each cell provide the linear, super-structural package of the genetic material (see genes, DNA)
CLL	Chronic lymphocytic leukaemia
CML	Chronic myeloid (or granulocytic) leukaemia
CNS	Central nervous system (brain, spinal cord)
DNA	Deoxyribonucleic acid. The basic chemical of which our genetic information is constituted — assembled into higher order units, gene and super-structures, chromosomes
EMF	Electro-magnetic fields. Non-ionizing radiation from pylons, electric cabling, electronic devices etc.,
FISH	Fluorescence *in situ* hybridisation. A labelling technique with fluorescent probes enabling scientists to visualise individual chromosomes or genes in single cells

Gene	The basic coding unit or block of genetic information in each cell. Some 20,000 to 30,000 genes exist in each human cell and most genes provide a chemical code for the synthesis of unique proteins — which are the functional workhorses of cells
Genome	A term for the total DNA information context of each cell's nucleus
Haematopoiesis	The production of all types of blood cells, mostly in the bone marrow in children and adults, but also in the liver in developing babies before birth.
Hickman line	An intravenous device inserted into patients for the repeated delivery of drugs and supportive measures such as blood, blood products and intravenous fluids
Leptomeninges	Soft envelope surrounding the brain and spinal cord
MRD	Minimal residual disease; a very sensitive molecular biology test (see PCR) for leukaemic cells that remain after treatment
PCR	Polymerase chain reaction. A technology that amplifies million of copies of genes (or small pieces of DNA) from single copies or small copy numbers. It has widespread application in biomedical sciences and forensic medicine
PKU	Phenylketonuria. Inborn defect in protein metabolism with excess of amino acid phenylalanine in the blood.
Platelets	Small particles of blood derived from megakaryocytic cells in the bone marrow; they prevent bleeding and easy bruising

Stem cell — A unique "primitive" cell type that serves as a founder to both generate and sustain huge numbers of progeny blood cells required each day. Responsible for both normal and leukaemic cell production

TPN — Total parenteral nutrition. Feeding by drip for patients who cannot take oral food and liquids

Translocation — An exchange of large units of genetic material, usually between two different chromosomes. Generates chimaeric chromosomes and chimaeric genes that play a key functional role in the development of leukaemic cells

T cell lineage — A major type of 'lymphoid' blood cell involved in the immunological defence against infection.

Index